The Future of Health: Emerging Technologies

David Priede, Ph.D.

The information included in this book is for educational purposes only. It is not intended or implied to be a substitute for professional medical advice. The reader should always consult a physician or healthcare provider to determine the appropriate information for their own situation or questions regarding a medical condition or treatment plan. Reading the information in this book does not constitute a physician-patient relationship. Some of the book's statements have not been evaluated by the Food and Drug Administration (FDA). The author and publisher expressly disclaim responsibility for any adverse effects that may result from the use or application of the information contained in this book.

Published and Printed in the United States of America.

BioLife Publishing
Weston
First Edition
10 9 8 7 6 5 4 3 2 1

Acknowledgments

So many people have been involved in the process of creating this book. I am grateful to all the participants who contributed to the many hours of planning, investigation, academic research, and studies that inspired this book. I also thank all my dedicated staff at BioLife Health Center and BioLife Neuroscience specially Larrie Hamilton and Milley Carrol for their leadership, continued support, and inspiration. Also, all my co-workers who provided their relentless guidance and input: Paisly Zenith, Danny Sullivan, Michelle Ryan, Cindy Hamilton, and Janet Anderson which I consider part of my family and feel grateful to have their dedication, knowledge, and wisdom. This book would have not been possible without the love and support of my parents and dearest friends.

I would like to send my deep appreciation and great consideration to the researchers, writers, editors and so many others who made this publication possible:

Researchers: Angela Zhang, Aditya Trivedi, Ashmita Reddy, Olivia Francis, Ian Zobrist, and Monique Srikijroj.

Statistics: Ashwin Jain.

Graphics Design: Elizabeth Croxon.

Editors: Sydney Antonoff-Wertheimer, Jhenna Becker, and Austin Oshima.

Senior Editor: Emma Foster.

Contents

Prologue

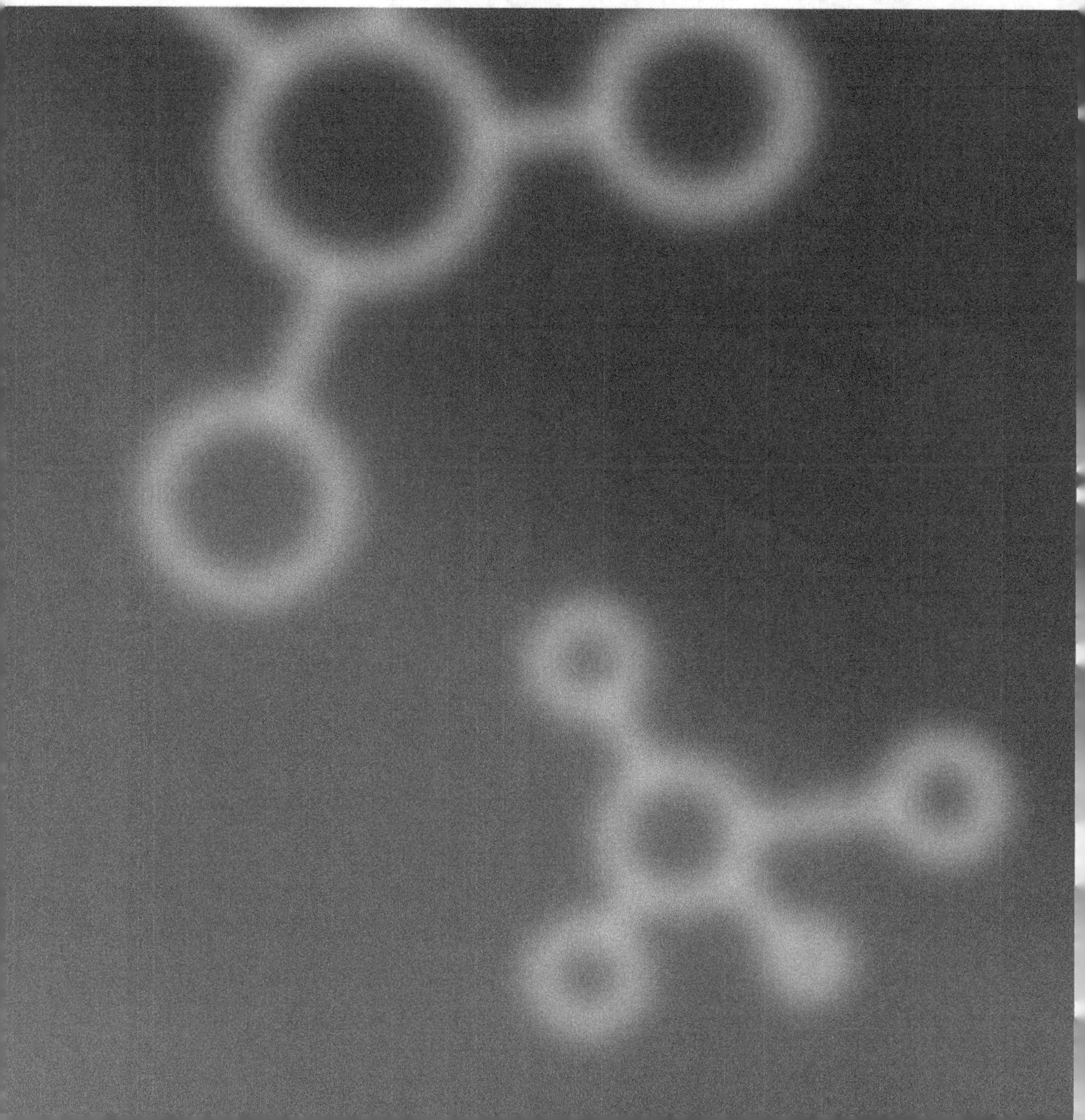

While no one knows what the future will bring, one can look at signs and the forces of change to start drawing a picture of the future of health. In essence, health will likely revolve around sustaining well-being rather than responding to illness. Prevention and early diagnoses driven by technological transformation will be central to the future of health. Interventions and treatments will be more precise, less complex and invasive, and more cost-effective. Health will be defined as an overall state of well-being, encompassing physical, mental, emotional, and social health. Healthcare is moving towards sustaining well-being rather than responding to illness. Technological healthcare advancements will increase preciseness and reduce complexness in healthcare while being more affordable.

Continuous monitoring will prove efficient in minimizing visits to the hospital and late discovery of diseases. Instant diagnosis and prescriptions delivered to your door will also be a part of the new primary care vision because these advancements will increase accessibility and affordability. Advancement in the utilization of health data will move us towards patient-centered, tailored, quality care, and patient engagement will be crucial for this transformation. The industry faces transformational changes, and spending will be dedicated to preventing and sustaining. Health treatments will shift from proactive and preventative to a more differential view of the patient. This means an increase in the precision of medicine being delivered, focusing more on the outcomes. The future of healthcare is at the tip of our fingers with these incoming technologies. As much literature has studied, patient-centered, evidence-based care is the most effective and efficient kind of care. Cutting-edge technologies will transform patient health by creating new approaches to prevention, early diagnosis, personalized treatment, continuous monitoring, and at home point-of-care. The new landscape includes improvements and advancements in virtual healthcare, artificial intelligence, nanomedicine, virtual and augmented reality, robot-assisted surgery, 3D printing, wearable healthcare trackers, medical tricorders, genome sequencing, and new drug development. These and other technological innovations will fundamentally change the nature of healthcare delivery by better connecting people with services, automating routine tasks, and analyzing patient health information to improve care decisions. New modalities and technologies will develop, breakthrough cures will occur, and healthcare organizations will shift priorities to patient needs.

Virtual Healthcare

Virtual healthcare is set to become a crucial aspect of delivering efficient and accessible healthcare in the future. The improvement in accessibility that virtual healthcare will provide is nearly endless. With minimal resources needed on the patient's end, virtual healthcare can transgress even the most remote and rural areas. Presently, emergency rooms are often filled with patients waiting for extended periods of time, but virtual healthcare helps reduce wait time to a fraction, keeping room in the ER for those who need it most. Particularly with the assistance of AI, assigning degrees of urgency nursing in the ER can be performed more efficiently, leading to a better flow in the emergency room. For instance, many youths find it an unnerving experience to get medical help in person, particularly when it comes to mental health. With virtual healthcare available to them without having to leave their home, it will and already has increased the number of people getting help. The growing aspect of virtual use in healthcare then expands the opportunities medical fields have for tackling various diseases and illnesses and technical problems plaguing healthcare today.

Artificial Intelligence (AI)

The self-service AI implementation is beneficial for patients because it has made obtaining care a more straightforward process. In terms of pharmaceuticals and medications, AI can help reduce the number of medication and dosing errors. These are human-made inaccuracies that often happen in the medical field, even with rules and regulations to prevent these errors from repeating. In the future, AI will outperform clinicians in these tasks. This will reduce error and increase patient satisfaction, safety, and costs. Additionally, in the field of medical imaging, AI is beneficial and efficient in analyzing symptoms. It will detect abnormalities faster than physicians as AI continues to be used and perfected. AI will also eventually be able to assist with tailoring individual care for each patient. This is a task that usually takes the work of several clinicians. However, with AI, hospitals and clinics can tailor and deliver patient-centered care more efficiently and effectively while reducing costs and human errors.

Brain-Computer Interfaces (BCI)

Brain-computer interfaces provide a direct communication pathway between an enhanced or wired brain and an external device. It measures the central nervous system and converts brain signals to electric signals to control and direct external medical devices such as personal computers, robotic arms, wheelchairs, and a person's muscles. It is widely beneficial for patients with neurological conditions and can be implemented in invasive and non-invasive methods. Passive BCIs allows for activities such as mental workload or affective states, and active BCIs uses brain strategies such as helping moving a limb. This technology is targeted to provide functionality for those with paralysis, and it is now being evaluated for other psychiatric disorders. Neurofeedback and BCIs can facilitate retraining brainwave patterns to treat disorders such as depression, anxiety, and ADHD.

Nanomedicine

Nanomedicine includes a wide range of applications, such as biosensors, tissue engineering, and diagnostic devices. Nanotechnology deals with the smallest components of the world's atoms and molecules. It can assist with navigating through parts of the body to search for disease, monitor the body, provide treatments and repairs, and regenerate the biological system. Past nanomedicine development includes small, smart pills for colon exams and other forms of small-scale, minimally invasive procedures. Nanotechnology is the system behind inventions meant to decrease lengthier procedures. These advances, such as smart patches, are highly beneficial for healthcare today, as traditional wound healing is time-consuming for the patients and constant manual checks and monitoring of the wound is not time-efficient for clinicians. Additionally, research on nanomaterials can lead to safer implants and stimulate cell growth. With further advancements in nanotech, these nanotechnologies will transform the monitoring and understanding of health, disease, and biology

Virtual and Augmented Reality

The inclusion of virtual and augmented reality in the training of clinicians and scientists is beneficial as virtual healthcare becomes more prominent, including therapy and immersive experiences. Training doctors and nurses may now be allowed to practice their skills before performing in a real-life situation. Clinical students want nothing more than a chance to practice their skills; however, these are not always the easiest to come across during their placements. When it does, there is pressure to perform for the first time on a real patient in front of several doctors. In addition, many students will also be able to perfect their skills and become accustomed to the routine of the tasks before performing them on a patient, mainly in fields of surgery or emergency situations.

Robotics and Robot-Assisted Surgery

Robotics has multiple uses in the healthcare field, from pharmabiotics, disinfectant robots, exoskeletons, robot companions, and surgical robots. Additionally, a telenursing robot allows nurses to control a robot to perform tasks with patients remotely. This will help with reducing physical workload, increasing accessibility, and alleviating emotional issues. Robots can assist with elderly care through companionship and possibly as an assistant in emergencies (such as calling for help). Rural areas heavily benefit from telenursing robots, as they can replace in person clinicians. Robot-assisted surgeries have allowed surgeons to perform on the body's narrowest and most minute locations, as these instruments are stunningly flexible and subtle. Robotic surgery also offers benefits for patients such as reduced discomfort, pain management, blood loss, risk of infection, and recovery time. Robots can also assist surgeons in physical tiredness during surgeries that require standing up for hours, such as urology surgeries.

3D Printing

3D printing is used in prosthetics, surgical cutting, and the creation of patient-specific bone, organs, and blood vessels.

Pharmaceutical companies have also utilized this technology with 3D printing pills containing several medicines in one. 3D printing aids in the creation of personalized prosthetics as well. This leads to shorter recovery times, the accuracy of treatments, and a more cost-efficient process. 3D printed anatomical models from patient-specific scan data are also a valuable tool for personalized care and precision in medicine. bioprinting (the construction, layer-by-layer, of a biological structures and organs) is a promising development, as it has already positively assisted surgeons by reducing complications and improving drug delivery.

Healthcare Trackers, Wearables, and Sensors

The development of wearable healthcare can aid in the development of health monitoring and non-invasive treatment. In the future, trackers, sensors, and other types of wearable devices will provide more accurate measurements beneficial for patients and clinicians alike. Patients will be able to monitor their health without attending doctor's appointments, and minor procedures will mean less recovery time. These types of processes will also be more cost-effective. Wearable devices are currently being studied to prevent and diagnose diseases, meaning patients will experience less time at the doctor's office and more time practicing healthier habits based on the data they collect and receive from these devices.

Medical Tricorders

A medical tricorder scans patients and shows their vital signs, health indicators, or diagnosis. It is a portable handheld device that is used to monitor patients. There are already similar devices measuring various medical parameters on the market right now. High-powered microscopes on smartphones that analyze for DNA abnormalities are already underway. These technologies can reduce physical workload, increase time efficiency, and provide better personalized care. Additionally, a digital first-aid kit can assist with discovering an infection early and send these remote diagnoses to physicians, saving time, costs and freeing the physicians to perform more demanding tasks.

Genome Sequencing

Genome science is predicted to revolutionize the diagnosis, prevention, and treatment of possibly all human diseases. It can assist with identifying diseases through the detection of abnormalities in the chromosome, where it then generates a genetic profile and produces targeted therapies. By 2030, genome sequencing will allow scientists to deeply analyze a single drop of blood, which can tell them what health issues DNA is predisposed to. It could end all permanent physical injuries and mental disorders. This can start at birth, where genome sequencing can be done and benefit those with rare diseases. Pharmacogenomics (tailor-made drugs adapted to an individual's genetic make-up) will refine diagnoses and guide better therapeutic approaches. With genome sequencing and other health technologies, better precision, and cost reduction within the healthcare system will be provided.

New Drug Developments

New techniques of drug developments can help with clinical trials, including new technologies such as chips lined with living human cells that reproduce blood and airflow as our bodies do. With this type of technology, new drugs can be tested on virtual patient models within minutes, saving time and cost in all areas of clinical research. AI has drastically lowered the time to create new medications and adopted by numerous pharmaceutical companies. Data sharing will substantially increase within the industry in the next few years. This will optimize the process, reduce time and costs, and increase safety. Virtual clinical trials will be able to take away the need for multiple study sites, lengthy trial periods and can reach a more significant number of participants.

The Neurobiopsychosocial Framework

This health framework acknowledges the impact of biological, psychological, and social factors on the state of one's overall health. The biological aspect identifies physiological alterations in overall health. The psychological part of the model reflects mood, personality, and behavior. The social element consists of environmental factors such as culture and socioeconomic status. The neurobiopsychosocial framework emphasizes the importance of the structure and functioning of the nervous system. The neurobiopsychosocial framework aims to analyze further the effects of the most complex and least-understood organ in the human body: the brain. The functions of the nervous system are thought by many to overlap in the biological, psychological, and social aspects of one's health, which further stresses the importance of the neurological factor. This new interdisciplinary model specifically analyzes how such factors play a role in health and illness.

Challenges

None of the new developments in healthcare, biotech, or other medical fields come without challenges and risks. Even with recent advancements, ethical practices need to be considered. Many products also need to be accurately tested to understand their limitations and how they can improve. New technologies such as AI, nanomedicine, or wearable trackers can ease clinicians' workload and diagnose patients faster and easier. Still, there is always a chance of error in the beginning stages of new tech products. Healthcare systems need to put patients at the center of their solutions and make healthcare convenient, accessible, and "user-friendly." This brings to light the need for healthcare organizations and professionals to embrace the digital realm. This is not only needed to understand pain points to address patient needs but to stay competitive. Contributing to the cause for concern, the aging population is far outpacing the entry rate of new healthcare providers in general, meaning the healthcare system is quickly approaching a crisis in which too few healthcare professionals are available to diagnose and treat patients. Now is the time to be bold in using new technologies, but it needs to be done safely, with patient safety and data security as top priorities. These changes could revolutionize healthcare. Looking at the new ways new emerging technologies can be implemented will give us insight into how we view our health.

Chapter 1

Emerging Health Technologies

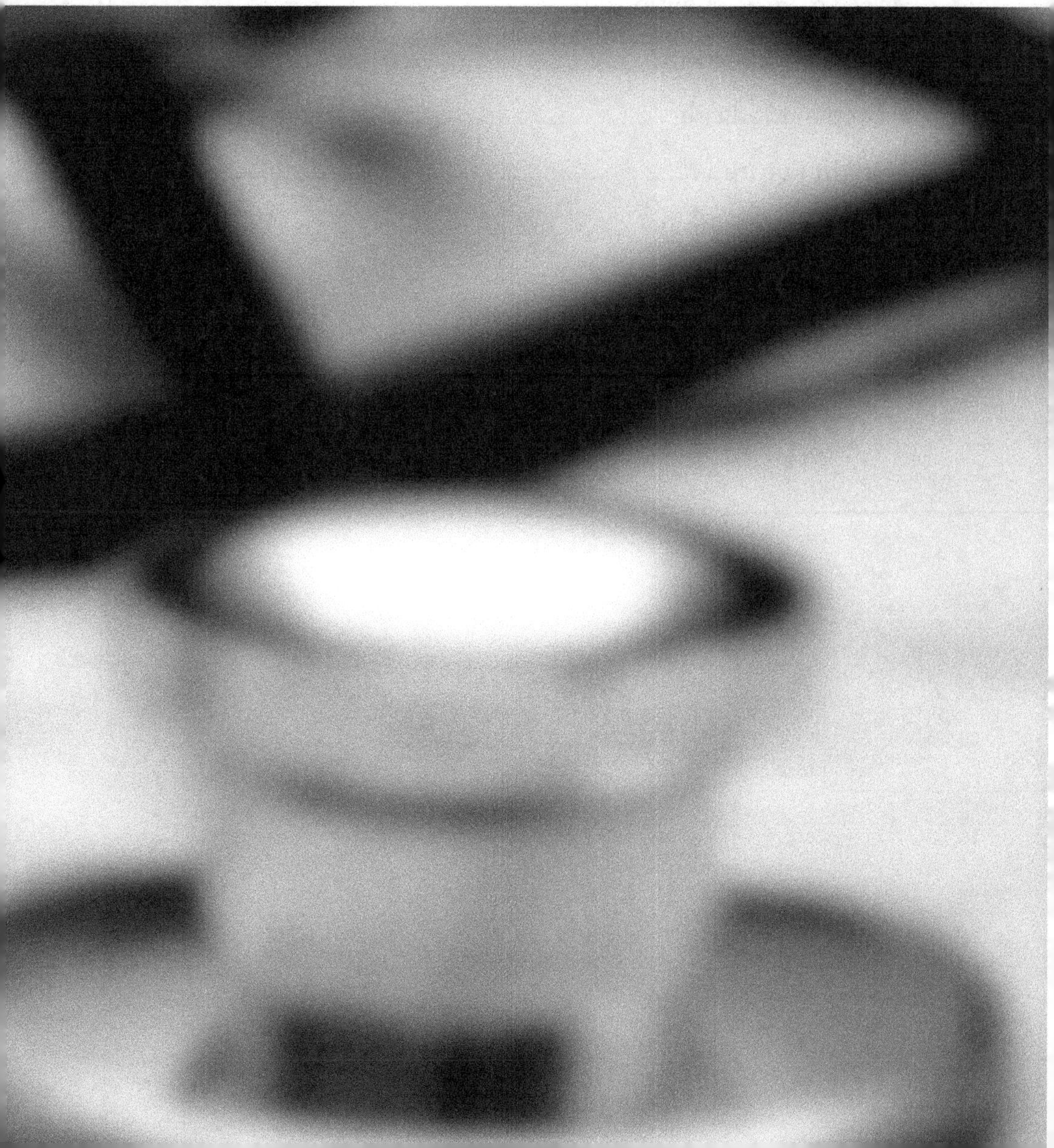

Contents

Introduction

Nothing is more important than good health. We all depend on the healthcare system and continue to interact with it throughout our lives. While no one knows what the future will bring, one can look at signs and the forces of change to start drawing a picture of the future of health. Many areas of change will collectively transform the existing health system from treatment-based reactionary care to prevention and well-being. The traditional limitations of the healthcare industry will fade out, and new roles, technologies, and procedures will emerge as exponential innovation drives the industry towards the future. Prevention and early diagnoses driven by technological transformation will be central to the future of health. Interventions and treatments will be more precise, less complex and invasive, and more economical. Health will be defined as an overall state of well-being, encompassing physical, mental, emotional, and social health.

A Look into The Future

Like many other sectors, healthcare is about to enter a period of rapid change. Longevity and the advance of new technologies, discoveries and innovative combinations of existing ones are among the many factors propelling patient empowerment, which is fundamentally changing how we prevent, diagnose, and cure diseases. The health care industry is on the brink of large-scale disruption. In the future, health will be defined by radically interoperable data, open yet secure platforms, and consumer-driven care. The exponential growth and advancement in healthcare and medicine will improve health, lower costs, and reduce geographic boundaries to access healthcare providers and specialists.

With emerging technologies, the digitalization of information will be the transformative force driving much of healthcare change. By 2040, health care as we know it today may no longer exist. There will be a fundamental shift from "health care" to "health." And while disease will never be eliminated, through science, data, and technology, we will be able to identify it earlier, intervene proactively, and better understand its progression to help pople more effectively and actively sustain their well-being. The future will be focused on wellness and managed by organizations that assume new roles to drive value in the transformed health ecosystem.

The development of advanced cognitive technologies will help analyze a patient's data and information for health insights. Streams of data will create a multifaceted and highly personalized picture of every individual's well-being. This data availability, with personalized AI, will enable accuracy and real-time interventions to get ahead of sickness and disease. The onset of illness, in some cases, could be delayed or eliminated as sophisticated tests and care take place at home.

Continuous Health Monitoring

Today, the proliferation of smartphones and the acceptance of wearable devices have emboldened medical devices and diagnostic companies to experiment with body-worn sensors that can monitor vital signs and transmit them in real-time to an online platform that can be remotely accessed. As medical technologies progress, health monitoring will become as common as smartphones.

Imagine someone who wakes up feeling sick. The person stands in front of the bathroom mirror. The mirror scans the body as an at-home diagnostic test instead of going to a clinic or physician's office to get a diagnosis. Open and secure data platforms connected to AI systems through virtual medicine would allow the patient to instantly get a diagnosis, order the necessary prescription, and deliver it to their home. With the advancements in technologies, a person can continuously monitor their health daily to identify risks earlier, so symptoms are identified, addressed, and prevented before getting sick.

Further in the future, the same bathroom mirror would perform a complete in-depth health evaluation. A prescription would not be needed because the person intervened before the onset of the illness. In both scenarios, individuals and families can address health issues at home while allowing physicians to focus on severe health conditions that require human intervention.

Sick Care vs. Prevention

The health industry is facing transformational changes. Technology and humans working together will result in remarkable achievements in healthcare. The U.S. healthcare system has begun to focus on wellness, but the overall approach remains focused on "sick care." Healthcare consumers typically only interact with the healthcare system when ill or injured. However, the future of wellness will be centered on well-being and prevention instead of treatment. Unlike now, healthcare will work transparently with the user instead of the organizations that drive the current U.S. healthcare system.

More healthcare spending will be devoted to sustaining health and preventing illness and less to assessing conditions and treating disease. Along with improving individuals' well-being and shifting the primary focus to identifying health risks and providing consumers ongoing advice and support, greater emphasis on well-being will result in fewer and less severe diseases. These, in turn, will reduce healthcare costs, allow reinvestment into new technologies, and expand the benefits to a much broader population.

Patient Engagement

Patient engagement is centered on providers and patients working together to improve health. A patient's greater engagement in healthcare contributes to improved health outcomes. Patients want to be engaged in their healthcare decision-making process, and those who are engaged in their care tend to be healthier and experience better outcomes. Patient engagement will become crucial for delivering high-quality services. While going through the analytics process, it is apparent that transparency in lowering costs and improving consumer habits is the key driving force for dynamic change.

An abundance of information is critical to driving commitment only if consumers are engaged. Consumers also need to understand new health models and make informed decisions. This information can become a catalyst for change when used with predictive tools. Additionally, beyond traditional risk assessment based on old-fashioned patient-reported outcomes, many medical sciences and technologies improve medical practice operations, reduce costs, and improve the patient experience. Patients are now starting to weigh their healthcare options in much the same way when buying a car or investing for retirement. They don't want decisions about their health to be made for them. Instead, they would prefer to learn more about their health from trusted sources and reach these decisions with their physician. This collaborative approach to healthcare helps health systems build trusted relationships, so patients stay invested in their care. Engaged patients are three times less likely to have unmet medical needs and twice as likely to seek care promptly when compared to unengaged patients.

The benefits of patient engagement include increased knowledge and understanding, encouraging patients to become actively engaged in their health, well-being, and healthcare choices, leading to improved care and fewer ER and physician's visits. In addition to improving care, patient engagement also has financial benefits as it reduces no-shows, aids in increasing revenue, and maintains a patient base. By collaborating and engaging with patients in the decision-making process, healthcare providers can make better decisions regarding a patient's health, improving the patient-provider relationship and overall patient retention. Physicians can better treat patients most effectively, ultimately becoming more time and cost efficient.

Proactive Medicine

Proactive means acting in anticipation of future needs and before the situation becomes a source of confrontation or crisis. In medical practice, it simply refers to the uncertainty of what could go wrong and measures to prevent or avoid it. Proactive medical care is a structured approach to care; it can influence how we think, manage and approach medical conditions. It can positively impact the way the medical community looks at and classifies diseases, the way we respond to clinical problems in hospitals, and the way we respond to the medical problem as society as a whole. The structured thought process and outcome-based practice preached by proactive medicine is the way to solve some of the health care systems. Focusing on crucial process improvements should pave the way toward the promotion of health systems.

Thanks to personalized health treatments, by 2035, the healthcare industry will have shifted from reactive to proactive and preventive medicine. This new era will encompass an integrated view of each person, where health could become a core value of our society. Virtual experience platforms will play a vital role in this transformation. With precision medicine being delivered on new healthcare platforms, individual patient value can be assessed, and the information used to engage policymakers in change. The objective is to create a new value-based model of care, focused less on the products and more on the outcomes.

A Bright Future

Cutting-edge technologies will transform patient health by creating new approaches to prevention, early diagnosis, personalized treatment, continuous monitoring, and “at home” point of care. The new landscape includes improvements and advancements in virtual healthcare, AI, nanomedicine, virtual and augmented reality, robot-assisted surgery, 3D printing, wearable healthcare trackers, medical tricorders, genome sequencing, and new drug development. These and other technological innovations will fundamentally change the nature of healthcare delivery by better connecting people with services, automating routine tasks, and analyzing patient health information to improve care decisions. New modalities and technologies will develop, breakthrough cures will occur, and healthcare organizations will shift priorities to patient needs.

Medical technology plays a massive role in the medical advancements we enjoy today. It has made the early and accurate diagnosis of diseases possible. We also have medical technologies to thank for innovative products and devices that help people survive and enjoy life as normally as possible. Additionally, modern medical technology has allowed telemedicine, with connected devices enabling users and medical practitioners to monitor their health. it's interesting to know where the industry stands. An excellent way to start is to examine medical technology statistics.

Just like in any industry, medical technology is not perfect. Even the most prominent companies face issues and threats. For example, almost half (45%) of health executives say rapid advancements in new technologies and scientific innovations can disrupt their industries. A considerable majority (88%) of medical technology executives rated advances in technology as a top challenge, followed by (63%) policy and regulatory activity and changes in consumer attitudes, behaviors, and spending. Furthermore, 54% of health executives say their employees will be challenged to figure out how to work with robots. Moreover, 75% of medical device industry players believe that having a better supply chain ability is a concern for the market. As supply chain costs account for 40% of the expenses found in the medical devices market today, improving performance in this area could boost profits for manufacturers by up to 20%.

Meanwhile, 70% of healthcare consumers are concerned about data privacy and commercial tracking associated with their online activities, behaviors, location, and interests. Furthermore, medical technology's significance became even more pronounced and recognized with the onset of the COVID-19 pandemic. As MedTech companies (Medical companies that use technologies products, services or solutions used to save and improve people's lives) continuously bring innovative and groundbreaking products to global health markets.

Statistics and Trends

- The global medical devices market size was estimated to be worth $447.63 billion in 2019. It is expected to grow to approximately $671.49 billion by 2027.
- The market is expected to grow at a yearly rate of 5.2% during the forecast period of 2020 to 2027.
- Analysis of the medical device market by country shows that the medical technology market size is dominated by the U.S., which accounts for 39%.
- The U.S. telemedicine market valuation is expected to reach $25.88 billion by 2027.
- At least 85% of health executives acknowledge that technology has become an inextricable part of the human experience.
- In general, medical technology companies spend approximately 21% of their annual revenue on research and development projects.

- 78% of health executives believe that the stakes for innovation have never been higher during and beyond COVID-19.
- 31% of MedTech leaders said reducing costs is the primary goal for their digital investments. Meanwhile, 25% say they invest to gain insights into the execution of business strategy, while another 25% invest to increase demand for their products. On the other hand, 19% say the investments are for improving the efficiency of their R&D process.
- At the beginning of 2020 (pre-COVID), 80% of physicians in the U.S. were not using virtual health in their patient interactions. Six months later, when COVID hit, about 85% of physicians increased their use of virtual technology, with 58% of them increasing usage by over 50%.
- It is estimated that by 2030, 2 in 3 healthcare visits will be virtual.
- The global internet-of-medical-things (IoMT) market accounted for $24.4 billion in 2019 and is expected to grow to $285.5 billion by 2029 at a yearly increase of 28.0%.
- In general, 56% of consumers will share their personal and health data to help with disease prevention, 45% to help the environment, 42% to help their community, 37% to help with problems such as crimes, and 35% to increase transparency.
- Around 71% of health executives believe robotics will enable the next generation of services in the physical world. Furthermore, 69% of healthcare organizations are piloting or adopting AI.

Chapter 2
Virtual Healthcare

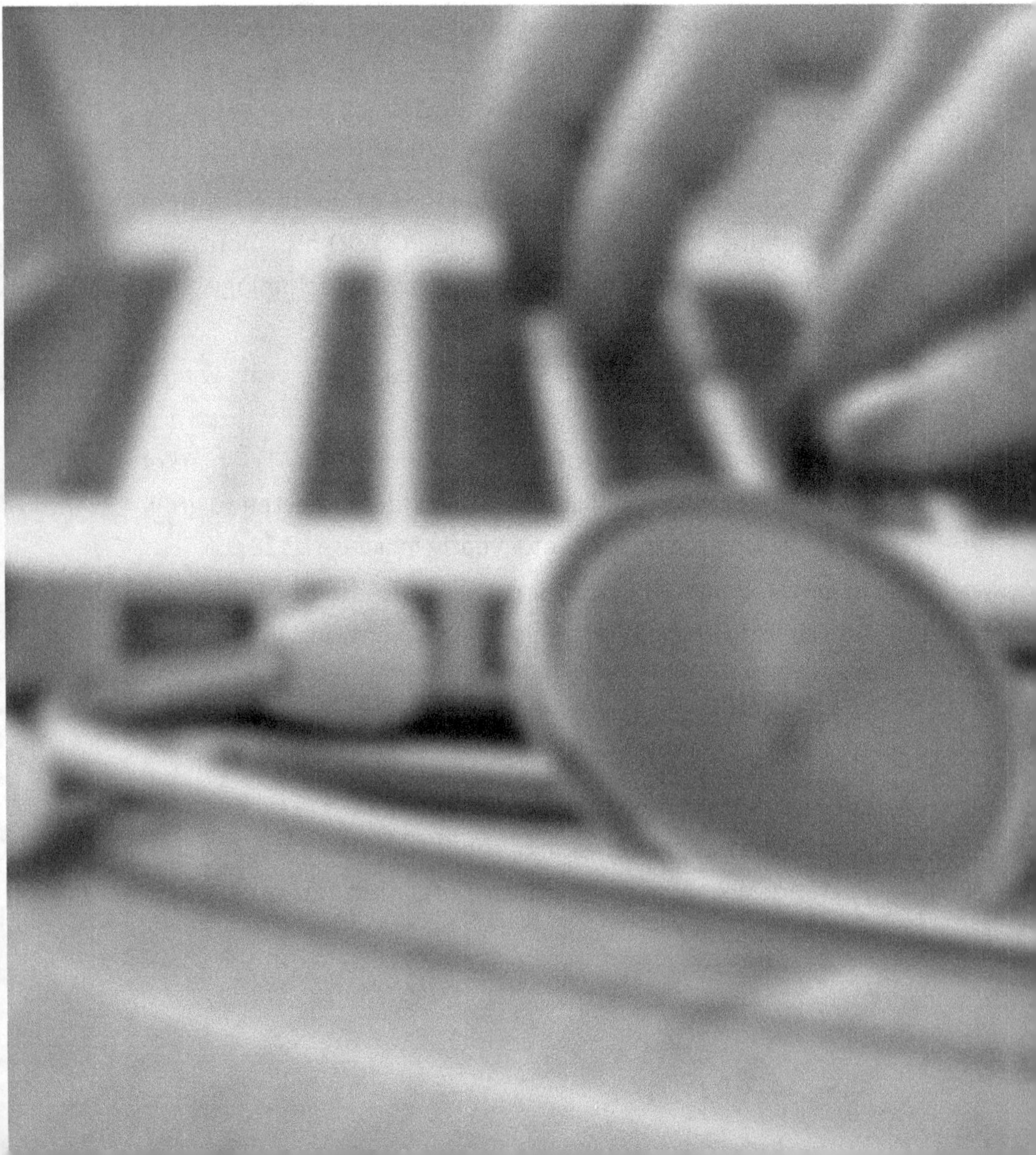

Contents

Introduction

At the beginning of the 20th century, radio revolutionized communications. Inspired by the rapid advancement in various fields, from entertainment to national defense, innovators soon began to imagine how doctors could serve patients through radio. In the 1940s, Pennsylvania transmitted radiographic images 24 miles between two cities via telephone lines. This was the world's first electronic medical record transmission example. In the 1950s, a Canadian doctor used this technology to build a tele radiology system used in Montreal and its surrounding areas. In the 1960s and 1970s, the U.S. Department of Public Health, NASA, the Department of Defense, and the U.S. Department of Health and Human Services invested ample resources in telemedicine research. Innovative projects such as STARPAHC (Space Technology for Advanced Healthcare in Rural Papagos Indian Reservation) have promoted research in medical engineering, leading to the rapid growth of telemedicine.

The telemedicine equipment used today is similar to early telemedicine equipment, but modern medical technology is smaller in size and has a broader range of functions. Fortunately, there are still many unknown areas in the telemedicine industry. Both private and government research companies have invested heavily in telemedicine, so this technology is developing almost faster than doctors can use it.

What is Virtual Healthcare?

With the advancement of technology, physicians can stay at the forefront of medical practice in more ways. With the rise of the digital age, significant improvements and innovations have been made in patient access, healthcare costs, and quality of care. One development that is expected to change the face of healthcare is "virtual healthcare" or "telemedicine." This is one or more methods by which doctors and other health care providers can communicate with patients without meeting them in person. This health care awareness is beneficial for patients who are too busy to go to an office or for people with limited mobility, transportation, or those living in remote areas. It can be used for online second opinions, doctor-to-doctor consultations, and family follow-ups. Virtual health services use technology to improve communication and information flow between patients, caregivers, and health care teams. Any interaction done remotely utilizing any form of communication is considered virtual care; this can include video sessions, text messages, phone calls, email, or any exchange of patient information between health professionals.

Virtual Healthcare Uses and Applications

Telemedicine connects patients with essential health services through video conferencing, remote monitoring, electronic consultation, and wireless communication. By increasing access to doctors and experts, telemedicine ensures service to patients in need. Currently, 76% of U.S. hospitals use video and other technologies to communicate remotely with patients and counseling professionals. Almost all state Medicaid and Medicare programs have some form of telemedicine service coverage as well as private insurance coverage for many of these services.

Looking to the future, virtual healthcare will continue to lay the necessary foundation for physicians and other medical personnel to provide patients with flexible care. Increasing patient participation will adopt digital-first strategies to reduce costs and make the entire experience more convenient for patients and caregivers. In the future, the combination of artificial and enhanced intelligence, home care, wearable devices, and two-way video will promote digital care.

Despite limited human resources, continued advances in AI will improve clinical insights. Nothing can replace knowledgeable and experienced caregivers; however, it could be effective if the information available to them increases and is more accurate. Continuous virtual observation of patients, data capture via wearable devices, and access to predictive algorithms can help providers foresee conditions that affect patient outcomes.

Additionally, accelerating telemedicine to provide proof of service to patients unable to see a doctor during pandemics is feasible and often the preferred option. Therefore, hospitals are looking for other ways to expand family health care participation. While this is primarily to reach patients who were isolated at home during the COVID-19 pandemic for example, it is also driven by the changing expectations of patients for easier access to care. The virtual care model represents the modern equivalent of past home visits. Technology platforms and various connected devices will become permanent elements in the household. These solutions provide a cost-effective way to reduce some of the expenses usually associated with hospitalization. Home care is an additional advantage in minimizing clinicians' chance of contacting patient's infections.

In addition, the proliferation of remote devices will also have an impact in the coming years. Healthcare trackers, sensors, and wearable devices such as smartwatches, fitness trackers, biosensors, electrocardiograms, and blood pressure monitors represent some of the first popular home devices. Remote technology that continuously measures and monitors patients' vital signs can accelerate providers' awareness of patient risk factors. By actively notifying healthcare providers of warning signs, clinicians can intervene earlier to prevent proliferation of conditions and illness. These interactive devices can also encourage patients to make better health decisions in real-time. The rise of these "digital medicine cabinets" technologies will provide providers with previously untapped ways to shift them from passive care to more proactive medical interventions.

Today, AI, home health, and wearable devices have achieved success, but the real power and benefits will come from combining them into an integrated ecosystem. In the past year, the use of telemedicine has reached an incredible level and established a new normal, which is expected to continue. This is the ideal time for suppliers to optimize these technologies and prepare for growth. The nursing room of the future will use video-enabled care to increase operational efficiency, improve the safety of employees and patients, and reduce differences in healthcare access.

During the COVID-19 pandemic, virtual health care became a vital tool. It can screen patients, provide low-risk and urgent care, virtual assist patients with physical therapy, virtual patient follow-up, etc. Before the pandemic, when it was necessary to treat patients from remote areas, it was required to shorten the waiting time in the hospital waiting room and waiting time for patients even doubled or tripled.

When preventive healthcare is needed, virtual healthcare will be used in the future. Virtual health also enables healthcare stakeholders and patients to share data and content and conduct personalized interactions remotely. This can provide convenient, high-quality care, thereby improving provider-patient interaction. Virtual robots and automation that support healthcare can help clinicians get rid of routine, clerical, and other repetitive tasks, giving physicians and other medical personnel more time to treat more patients. For example, virtual assistants can manage appointments, prescriptions, and electronic medical records.

With virtual healthcare and telemedicine, patients do not need to drive to the doctor's office, park their car, walk inside, and sit in the waiting room when they are sick. They can see a doctor from their home or office. Virtual tours can more easily adapt to busy schedules. Patients may not need to miss work or arrange childcare services with telemedicine. Looking to the future, the critical challenge may be optimizing the use of telehealth. All signs point to more health at home and determining how to optimize in-person and virtual care.

The Future of Virtual Healthcare

Today, doctors use virtual healthcare to make phone calls or video calls to consult their patients. A survey of approximately 1,600 health care providers found that due to their experience during the COVID-19 pandemic, nearly 70% of people are motivated to use telemedicine more often than personal visits. More than half said their outlook is due to health and service improvement. The survey was conducted in July and August by the COVID-19 Healthcare Alliance Working Group, which consists of the American Medical Association, American Telemedicine Association, Change Healthcare, Digital Medicine Association, Mayo Clinic, and the Massachusetts Health Quality Partners. The formation of Mass Challenge Health Tech and MITRE has increased efforts to continue to expand telemedicine by permanently establishing emergency measures designed to help providers during a crisis. Over 75% of respondents said that telemedicine helps them provide quality care to patients. The strong support shown for telehealth, as evidenced in these results, reinforces the knowledge that telehealth is critical to how we deliver healthcare today. The use of telehealth during the COVID-19 pandemic highlights its importance in care delivery. Its continued use will be instrumental in connecting to patients everywhere.

There are three main benefits of using virtual healthcare in the future. The first is to provide better access to people. Telemedicine appointments are especially promising for patients living in rural areas, given the lack of qualified providers in many of these areas. Virtual healthcare can provide healthcare services to millions of people across the country and elsewhere.

The second benefit is that the cost of medical care is reduced. Virtual healthcare awareness can save $6 billion annually. Better chronic disease management, shared health professionals, reduced travel time, and shorter hospital stays are a few of the savings. The top benefit of implementing virtual healthcare in the medical field is improving care. Telemedicine can improve the quality of care and patient visits without affecting safety. You can strengthen the relationship with the patient's doctor and expand the scope of visits. Additionally, clinicians want to know with certainty that their diagnosis, prognosis, and treatment are rooted in evidence-based practice; patients want to have confidence in their providers' expertise.

Telemedicine tools can solve these problems. For example, the virtual assistant can listen to the conversation between the provider and the patient, look up the latest evidence-based practice related to the patient's condition in the digital clinical guide library, and summarize key findings to help the provider give advice. This will allow the physician to focus on their patients. Portable and remote devices can help clinicians measure patient health indicators. After the consultation, the virtual assistant can prepare comprehensive and straightforward discussion content, recommended treatment methods, and summaries of related research articles for the physician to view. After the physician has reviewed the material, the patient can receive the content safely through an encrypted messaging system.

Risks and Challenges

There are many challenges in implementing virtual healthcare in the medical field. Bandwidth issues, access through a range of devices, integration into an organization's technological infrastructure, addressing HIPAA compliance, and other security considerations. In addition, payment systems, misdiagnosis, and widespread implementation are some of the main problems.

There is no guarantee of parity between telemedicine and face-to-face medical care regarding costs. In the 28 states that passed pay equality laws, there are no agencies to enforce these laws. This may hinder the role of telemedicine in reducing health care costs and expanding the scope of services. It may also prevent providers from providing telemedicine because comparable payments cannot be guaranteed. As for misdiagnosis, which usually occurs in face-to-face medical care, the risk of misdiagnosis in telemedicine is greater.

HIPAA compliance and platform reliability and security are common apprehensions of providers and their medical computer systems. Some providers may even assume they can use existing communication platforms such as Facetime or Skype to communicate with colleagues and patients. It helps if all involved understand the need for, and value of, a safe and secure communication platform which complies with the required HIPAA laws national standards to protect sensitive patient health information from being disclosed without the patient's consent or knowledge.

The challenges of the widespread implementation of telemedicine involve many different fields because "telemedicine" can refer to many different things, from robotics to telephone consultation. Exceeding the healthcare industry's benchmarks and regulations is critical for healthcare organizations seeking to deliver virtual care and ensure security, privacy, and compliance.

Summary

The awareness of telemedicine in health care is beneficial for patients who are too busy to go to a physician’s office, can’t leave their home or live in rural areas. By increasing access to doctors and experts, telemedicine ensures that patients receive the proper care. Currently, 76% of U.S. hospitals use video and other technologies to communicate remotely with patients and counseling professionals. Almost all state Medicaid and Medicare programs have some form of telemedicine service coverage, and private payers are receiving coverage for many telemedicine services as well.

Looking to the future, virtual healthcare will continue to lay the necessary foundation for doctors to provide patients with flexible care. Increased patient participation will adopt digital-first strategies to reduce costs and increase convenience. Despite limited human resources, continued advances in artificial intelligence will improve more convenient clinical insights and serve more patients.

Continuous virtual observation of patients, data capture via wearable devices, and access to predictive algorithms to help providers predict conditions that affect patient outcomes will collectively improve care. The virtual care model represents the modern equivalent of past home visits.

These solutions provide a cost-effective way to reduce some of the expenses usually associated with hospitalization and offer greater convenience and comfort for patients. There is an additional advantage of home care, which is to minimize the chance of clinicians contacting infected patients. Remote technology that continuously measures and monitors patients' vital signs can accelerate the provider's awareness of patient risk factors. By actively reminding healthcare providers of warning signs, clinicians can intervene earlier to prevent adverse or catastrophic events and provide patients with the correct care.

These interactive devices can encourage patients to make better health decisions in real-time. In the past year, the use of telemedicine has reached an incredible level and established a new way to offer healthcare. The nursing room of the future will use video-enabled care to increase operational efficiency, improve the safety of employees and patients, and reduce differences in healthcare access to all. Virtual health also enables healthcare, stakeholders, and patients to share data and content remotely and conduct personalized interactions.

Telemedicine appointments are especially promising for patients living in remote rural areas. Given the lack of qualified providers in many of these areas, virtual healthcare can be a lifesaver. Virtual healthcare can provide healthcare services to millions of people across the country. The ultimate benefit of implementing virtual healthcare in the medical field is that it improves the quality of care and reduces time and costs.

Statistics and Trends

- Telehealth isn't a new idea or need. Home-based medical care was mentioned as early as 1879 in a Lancet article about using the telephone to reduce unnecessary office visits.
- More than 60% of physicians reported that telehealth is easy to use within their practice across urban, suburban, and rural locations.
- Most telehealth use were for adults aged 18–49 years (43% in 2020 and 69% in 2022).
- More than 50% of physicians reported improved satisfaction with their work while using telemedicine.
- 68% of physicians reported that they wanted to increase the use of telehealth in their practice.
- While most midsize to large employers offer a telemedicine benefit, about 9% of eligible employees use it.

- Costs associated with eldercare needs are expected to strain the healthcare system. The vast majority of older adults are open to telemedicine, despite assumptions that they would be less willing to use technology.
- Telehealth surveys found telemedicine satisfaction to be very promising as 42% were extremely satisfied, 36% were somewhat satisfied, 16% were neutral, 4% not satisfied, and 2% extremely dissatisfied.
- 79% of patients say that scheduling a telemedicine follow-up visit is more convenient than arranging an in-person follow-up.
- 40% of millennials say that a telemedicine option was “extremely or very important.” Numbering 83 million, millennials now comprise the largest segment of today’s workforce. Millennials place a high value on both ensuring convenience and limiting treatment costs.
- The use of telemedicine has been shown to allow for better long-term care management and patient satisfaction.
- Net cost employer savings is estimated at $19-$121 per telemedicine visit.
- Over the last decade, average premium contributions by employers have increased 51%, from $10,008 to $15,159. Increasing the use of telemedicine can reduce costs by 31% on average.
- More than half (53%) of patients say they left a scheduled doctor’s appointment because the office wait was too long.
- Rural dwellers face more significant barriers to accessing good mental healthcare. 65% of nonmetropolitan counties do not have a psychiatrist, and nearly half do not have a psychologist.

- 93% of patients report that they would use telemedicine to manage prescriptions.
- 91% say telemedicine would help them stick to appointments, manage prescriptions and refills, and follow regimen recommendations.
- Telemedicine decreased mortality and length of stay in the ICU.
- Reported hospital mortality decreased from 13.8% before telemedicine to 11.8% after telehealth implementation.
- 62% of survey respondents paid an average of $1 to $30 out-of-pocket per telehealth visit.
- Insurance or Medicare and Medicaid completely covered telehealth services for 63% of respondents to a national survey.

Chapter 3
Artificial Intelligence

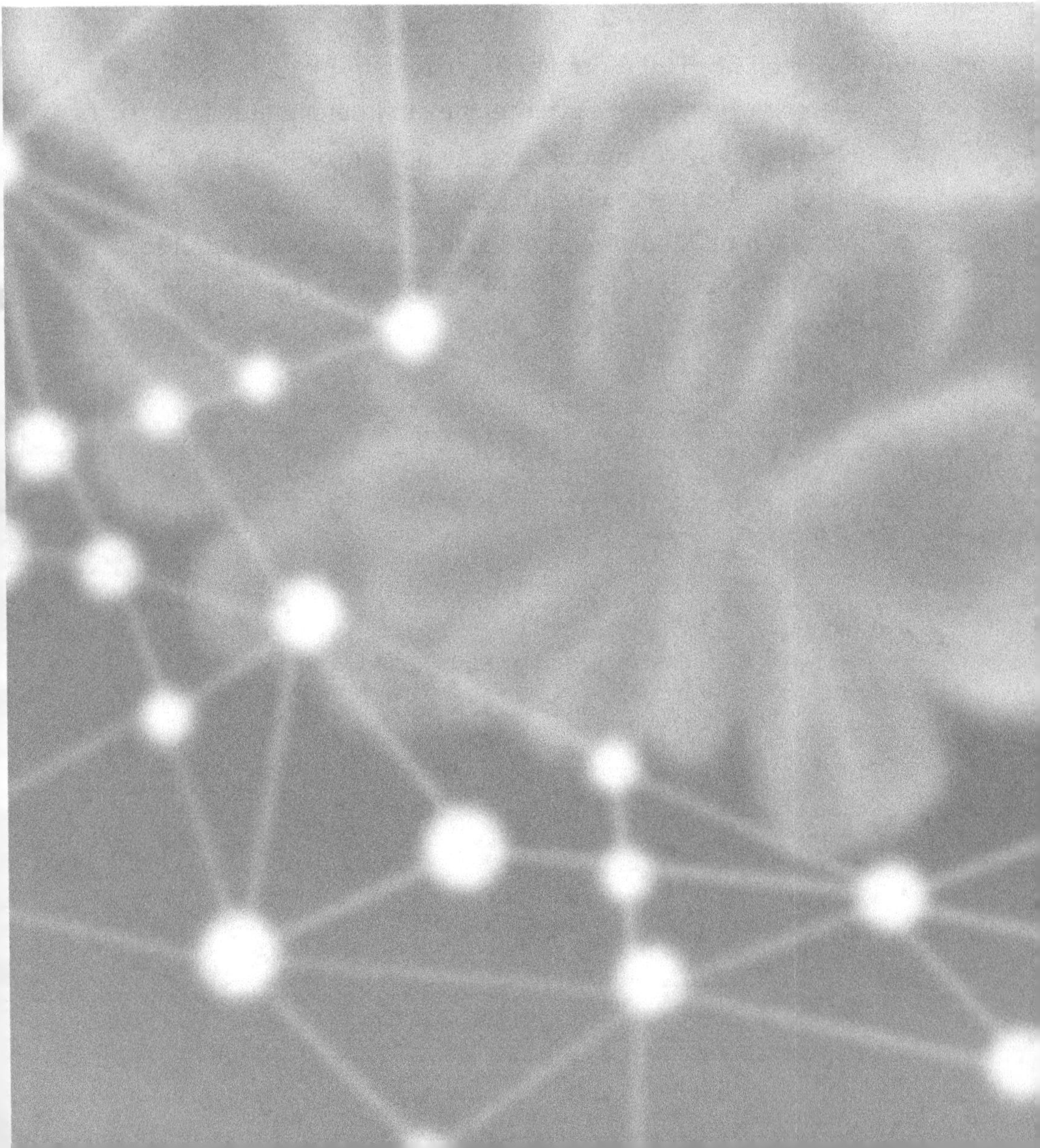

Contents

Introduction

The concept of artificial intelligence (AI) originated in the 1950s when a British mathematician and logician questioned if machines could think. In the early 1970s, AI was considered to have potential applications in the healthcare industry and started being applied to biomedical problems. AI was then slowly incorporated into clinical settings in the following decades. Extensive research later concluded that hybrid intelligent systems were among the new uses of AI in healthcare. As this technology has progressed, deep neural networks (deep neural networks use sophisticated mathematical modeling to process data in complex ways) have shown performances on par with human experts for many tasks.

In addition, several AI systems derived from the first problem-solving program, "Dendral." This program can identify infectious bacteria and provide the respective dosage of antibiotics required to destroy them through data analytics. Because of these earlier developments in AI, further development in healthcare was possible. AI could apply algorithms to accommodate sparse data and conquer new levels of assessment techniques required in healthcare. With these developments in AI, the applications in the healthcare industry are limitless. It is crucial to have a thorough understanding of AI.

What is AI?

AI has revolutionized many elementary processes humans perform manually by automating the process through computer networks and technologies. AI has already taken over assembly-line processes, jobs of factory workers, phone operators, telecommunication, customer service, and cashiers as well in other parts of the world as humans are being taken over by robots and AI and these are just to name a few. Another critical purpose of AI is to utilize and exploit the potential of computer-based technologies to do more ambitious jobs and ease the lives of humans.

Whether these three functions of AI are used individually or in unison, their applications in healthcare and medicine are limitless. It is anticipated that AI technologies will continue to progress faster in healthcare's future, potentially completely redesigning and revolutionizing this industry. They will be able to perform tasks that range from simple chatbots to complex computer-aided detection (CAD) systems for reading imaging data to analyze and diagnose diseases. One of the most anticipated applications of AI in healthcare is its potential to improve provider and physician productivity and quality of care, enhance patient involvement, and improve patient access to healthcare. AI in healthcare also holds the potential to refocus patient care and healthcare on prevention, awareness, and well-being.

AI can modify the healthcare field to improve the efficacy of current practices and shift the healthcare methodologies used today to focus more on patient care. AI can use algorithms (a process to be followed in calculations or other problem-solving operations by a computer) to enable healthcare workers, physicians, and hospitals to analyze patient data and develop therapies and treatment plans tailored toward the patient's specific genome (a complete set of DNA). AI possesses the potential to recognize patterns to the extent that it would be able to diagnose patients and determine which treatment plan will yield the best outcome for an individual. For instance, supercomputers running on AI will be used to develop therapies from a database of molecular structures for safe, existing medicines that could be redesigned to treat current and future viruses. AI's algorithms would outperform human physicians to identify conditions and improve costs and outcomes.

AI Uses and Applications

Experts in AI predict that networked artificial intelligence will serve as a medium for human efficiency, increase convenience in day-to-day lives, and reduce errors and costs in various tasks. The principal goal of AI is to transform the way people interact, pull together information, and obtain goods and services. In healthcare, AI can also use speech recognition, like voice assistants, to interact with patients and families in lobbies and waiting rooms to help physicians and practitioners prioritize their time and focus more on treatments and solutions.

While each AI technology alone can contribute substantial value, the potential lies in the synergies generated through use with diagnoses, treatment, and ongoing health maintenance. In patient self-service, patients can efficiently schedule appointments, pay bills, and fill out or update forms. This application of AI in healthcare shows that AI will modernize patient self-service, increasing cybersecurity and minimizing cybercrimes. It will provide the necessary analytics and threat identifications that cybersecurity professionals can use to reduce breach risk and improve patient's data security. Implementing self-service programs helps hospitals get benefits such as reduced patient waiting times, fewer errors, manageable payment options, reduced cost, and increased patient satisfaction. Provider organizations are gradually developing interactive online portals with chatbots for patients to complete these activities, medication refills, and simple administrative tasks. In our day-to-day lives, we have already begun to see the positive impact of voice assistants, which can also be applied to healthcare. Current implementations such as virtual health assistants (VHAs), chatbots using NLP (processing and analyzing large amounts of human language), concept extraction, and analysis technologies are all used to create an interactive patient experience. This will help healthcare workers prioritize their patients and their practice rather than engaging in tasks that hinder their ability to deliver care and service to the individual in question.

In the future, advances in AI will likely generate additional capabilities for CAD solutions. Over time, it would not be surprising to see the accuracy of imaging studies exceed that of radiologists, and neurologists with CAD systems potentially becoming the primary interpreters of imaging studies. A recent study explored the hindering and facilitating factors of CAD solutions and AI applications in radiology and brain imaging. The report concluded that for AI applications will improve the quality of clinical radiology and brain imaging. This conclusion is evidence of the clinical added value of AI applications and shows just how significant the potential of AI can be. AI will allow physicians to review imaging studies that exceed a certain level of uncertainty of the CAD/AI system. In addition, dermatology also uses CAD to help diagnose skin lesions at high risk of cancer. CAD dermatology systems learn about the various appearances of dermatological conditions by reviewing several images of lesions and diagnoses. Another recent study concluded that a CAD system showed 80% for classifying 23 diseases in the dermatology field. With AI, a physician and their team can build an advanced medical data model and then use AI and machine learning to adapt it to each person's profile.

As of now, AI is being implemented in healthcare, labor, inequality, and ethics. In these applications, AI serves a clear purpose: to end inequality and ethically execute all operations and functions. AI is used in situations where efficiency is being compromised. An example of this is when labor workers cannot prioritize their tasks because of their overwhelming workload. In this situation, AI's ability to automate labor work will help healthcare workers improve effectively in the work environment.

Another instance where AI is challenged during times of inequality and ethics is the COVID-19 pandemic. Because of the fears of contracting the coronavirus, many individuals opted out of visiting their local clinics and their family physicians, yielding a decreased quality of health. With the implementation of AI, virtual meetings with physicians were set up at an efficient rate. Individuals and families unable to afford any form of transportation to their local clinic can exploit the potential of AI by using their electronic devices to connect with their family physicians. However, AI health chatbots are focused more on efficiency and effectiveness than actual patient experience and care. For these AI chatbots to be used to their full potential in healthcare, they must be centered on the user and address patients' concerns.

In the future, AI has many application possibilities to be integrated into management and leadership in the healthcare industry. AI has already benefited workers because it can facilitate complex jobs and increase productivity. In the coming years, it is predicted that roughly 50% of the current work in the healthcare sectors can be automated with technologies that exist today. The tasks that healthcare workers perform can also be automated. For instance, image processing, data analytics, report summaries, scheduling, prescribing, drug preparation, and vaccine development could be automated. When and where AI will come in handy is only something time will tell, but as of now, it is predicted that when there is room for improvement, there is room for AI.

AI has already been integrated into various tech, automation, and manual labor businesses. However, AI is also revolutionizing the education systems to increase the convenience of education healthcare workers and students. School systems have already begun using AI to help develop skills in students and advance their testing. The primary goal of AI in education is to create a personalized and adaptable learning environment for students. A typical application for AI in both teaching and healthcare is universal accessibility. AI has the potential to provide global classrooms for students worldwide at a fraction of the cost. AI can serve as their translator eliminating language barriers for students of different ethnicities. AI can reduce the need for human translators in the healthcare industry and re-invest its resources into futuristic technologies. AI is already being used in hospital settings to help schedule appointments with physicians worldwide and is resulting in easier patient access to their physicians regardless of location.

AI is already in the office, transforming how people interact, consume information, and obtain goods and services. It has already been integrated into the automation industry and has begun automating administrative tasks. Booking appointments, house showcases, interviews, enrollment processes, and essential multiple-choice evaluations are all examples of basic administrative tasks that AI has tackled. And these are just a few of the applications of AI in the present day; the future applications of AI are still being researched.

AI's predictive functions are the most common applications in the healthcare field. These tools are likely to influence future urban health policies internationally. Companies use their predictive AI technologies to anticipate COVID-19 in China before it caught the rest of the world in late 2019. AI applications aim to reduce the time in viral detection and use AI to enhance global data communication across information systems. Early detection of viruses can prevent global pandemics and give a head start to vaccine development.

AI's pattern recognition capabilities will change the healthcare business field entirely, remodel the process of investing, and reinvent healthcare and well-being. Business owners and entities can see more detailed reports of consumer behaviors and plan their business processes accordingly. Investors can see likely outcomes of their investments and make wiser healthcare decisions based on patterns forecasted by AI. AI will accelerate the rate of developing new pharmaceutical treatments and personalize medical therapies by leveraging analytics to "mine" previously untapped sets of information of clinical data details.

The Future of AI

Today, many radiologists and other healthcare physicians use AI to improve their day-to-day practices more efficiently. For instance, by mobilizing fundamental AI and deep learning applications in medical imaging, the way future generations will access healthcare will be redefined. There are currently many applications of AI in epidemiology (the study of distribution and determinants of health-related states and events in specified populations.) Epidemiologists now use AI primarily for data analytics and extensive scientific research and reporting to reach informative and enlightening conclusions in the healthcare field. These are just some of the present-day applications of AI. In the future, there will be more applications and integration of AI into most healthcare systems.

The increasing popularity and demand for AI started from the vision that AI would help people in ways humans cannot. AI has the potential to revolutionize healthcare and medical practices. AI can reduce costs and offer new possibilities for public transport, education, waste, and energy management. Numerous AI applications can make humans' lives more sustainable and environmentally conscious.

AI is very cost-effective as an investment that will reduce healthcare costs significantly. AI's impact through natural language processing (NLP) and machine learning (ML) transforms healthcare delivery. Beyond health assistants, NLP and ML are used as part of other patient-oriented functions. For instance, visual image applications verify that patients have taken their correct medications. Rather than having to pay individuals to monitor the patients or regular patient check-ups, AI can use this visual image identification function to reduce employment costs in the healthcare field and optimize patient experience and the convenience of the healthcare workers and the patients. For clinicians, AI will offer more effective diagnosis and treatment tools. For instance, in imaging, AI is presently being used in computer-aided detection, or CAD systems, to retrospectively learn how different clinical abnormalities show up in imaging studies by analyzing both image data and related clinical information. This means that physicians will be able to focus more on executing the treatment plan rather than investing their time in finding the correct diagnoses and appropriate treatment plans. After reviewing many images and associated clinical data to achieve an adequate level of learning, CAD systems use the knowledge to identify areas of abnormality in imaging prospectively. CADs can generate a differential diagnosis (a procedure that differentiates between two or more conditions behind an individual's symptoms). For radiologist assessment, CAD is currently used for various imaging studies, including mammography, to identify areas suspicious of breast cancer.

One of the biggest reasons AI is important in the field of healthcare is because of its preventive applications for diseases Researchers successfully created an algorithm that predicts and forecasts coronary heart assaults in patients at a more effective and quicker rate than many experienced physicians using traditional guidelines. This capability of AI can help physicians tackle diseases and patient cases before the matter reach an irreversible stage or a state where life can only be prolonged. Through the power of machine learning and its intuitive nature, AI can reduce costs in the healthcare field. AI has the potential to make the industry more cost-effective, improve the quality of results from laboratory results, and grow more effective in detection, diagnostics, and treatment development.

Risks and Challenges

One of the most pressing ethical challenges of AI in healthcare is the question, "How will the use of AI to assist patients' care interface with the principles of informed consent?" Informed consent is when the physician gives the patient information about a treatment plan, including the risks and benefits. Informed consent is established to ensure that the patient has all the information to decide their health. The ethical challenge with the application of AI in healthcare asks to what extent physicians and clinicians are responsible for educating the patient about integrating AI into their treatment plan. Typically, physicians would not break down the software and hardware components of equipment that will be involved in a patient's treatment plan; however, because AI uses ML and data inputs, the question is, "Do physicians have a responsibility to inform patients about AI being integrated into the equipment being used?"

In addition, questions about the safety and transparency of AI used in healthcare have increased and posed one of the most significant ethical challenges for AI. For example, an AI software for oncology reportedly gave unsafe recommendations for cancer treatment. It was later revealed that the problem was in the training of the software. The input it was being fed was not actual patient data but rather a few synthetic cancer cases devised by a group of physicians. As of now, there is no concrete way to ensure that AI keeps it promises. A large portion of this problem stems from the basic concept of AI systems, which is that the output is solely dependent on its input. Algorithmic fairness and biases are a subcategory of this challenge of AI in healthcare. The human-trained algorithm ML system will only be as trustworthy, effective, and fair as the data it provides and trains. In other words, if the input is not valid and comes from synthetic or partially transparent datasets, then the output of the AI can potentially cause more harm than good in the healthcare industry.

Another example is an AI app that aims to help diagnose and detect acute kidney injury, recently raised concerns about data privacy for technological solutions. This was harmful to AI implementation in healthcare, though the app did not use AI. Ultimately, if patients do not trust AI, its integration and sustainability in healthcare will fail. All in all, the data's ownership and use must be kept under the doctor-patient policy and HIPPA compliant laws. The patient's privacy is given the utmost importance when it comes to data handling, processing, and analysis. However, the biggest challenge with AI is how much trust can be put into it with these confidentiality and data privacy policies.

Summary

AI will revolutionize the world's industries to optimize our current living patterns. The situations where AI can be integrated are limitless using machine learning (ML), deep learning (DL), and the three different applications of AI. Ranging from simple cognitive engagement such as virtual reality to something as complex as surgery, AI has the potential to modernize many of the processes individuals currently perform. AI aims to ease and better individuals' lives and integrate itself in ways that will serve and benefit humanity.

We, as individuals, have already integrated simple and complex AIs into our day-to-day lives. For instance, many individuals in today's world who possess smart devices use voice assistants to execute simple tasks around their environment. Search engine optimization or tailored ads are two of the most passive uses of AI that most of the world's population uses without recognizing that they are using AI. But this is just the beginning of who is using AI. We currently use it as individuals, but eventually, the healthcare industry will continue to further integrate AI processes into their activities. The healthcare industry will likely allow AI to interact with their patients more frequently and permit AI to execute specific treatment plans. And of course, AI has the potential to create a vast global network that will remove many of the barriers faced by individuals today.

AI is being applied worldwide, from something as simple as elementary video games to something as complex as aviation control and vehicle control. Specifically, many hospitals and healthcare industries have begun opting into AI integration practices. In inefficiency, sustainability, and reliability cases, AI is implemented to rectify the situation and ensure that tasks and operations are executed cost-effectively. AI will be used in the future when essential integration can allow for an optimized user experience.

In conclusion, AI will revolutionize most industries and new industries that may exist in the future. The healthcare industry will be reinvented in a way centered around AI and efficiency to focus more on prevention and well-being. With the integration of AI in the healthcare industry, physicians, clinicians, and other healthcare providers will be able to focus more on patient care and well-being rather than on diagnosing the patients and developing a treatment plan. Scientists worldwide will have complete access to datasets that will make vaccine development a much quicker and efficient process to the extent that diseases can be cured and treated before they spread. AI has been changing the healthcare industry already, and by overcoming the few challenges that are known today, AI has the potential to improve the practices and operations of every sector, especially healthcare.

Statistics and Trends

- AI technology can use software algorithms to complete tasks that require human intelligence.
- AI will affect research and development, billing, and digitized supply chain.
- When combined, key clinical health AI applications can potentially create $150 billion in annual savings for the U.S. healthcare economy by 2026.
- Unlike legacy technologies that are only algorithms/tools that complement a human health AI today can truly augment human activity.
- AI is exploding in popularity. Growth in the AI health market is expected to reach $9.6 billion by 2026, a compound annual growth rate of 40%. In just the next five years, the health AI market will grow more than 10x.
- Acquisitions of AI startups are rapidly increasing. The health AI market is set to increase by 40% through 2025.
- AI is already being used to detect diseases, such as cancer, more accurately and in their early stages. The use of AI enables the review and translation of mammograms 30 times faster with 99% accuracy, reducing the need for unnecessary biopsies.
- The proliferation of consumer wearables and other medical devices combined with AI is also being applied to oversee early-stage heart disease, enabling doctors and other

caregivers to better monitor and detect potentially life-threatening episodes at earlier, more treatable stages.

- Drug research and discovery is one of the more recent applications for AI in healthcare. By directing the latest advances in AI to streamline the drug discovery, there is the potential to significantly cut both the time to market for new drugs and their costs.
- Big data could save medicine and pharma up to $100B annually as a result of improved efficiencies in clinical trials and research, better insight for decision-making, and new tools that will help insurers, regulators, physicians, and consumers make better decisions.
- Machines are now learning how to read CT scans and other imaging diagnostics tests to identify abnormalities. Although some predict the end of radiologists as we know them, and others see AI acting as a radiologist's assistant.
- AI is already being used by the pharma industry in the initial screening of drug compounds, as well as to determine what drugs might work better for individuals based on their DNA.
- There have already been some powerful indicators of AI's influence to help monitor and predict health epidemics around the world and, in one case a computer algorithm identified an Ebola outbreak nine days before the World Health Organization reported it.
- Artificial intelligence and machine learning in healthcare will continue to get better and impact disease prevention and diagnosis, extract more meaning from data across various clinical trials, help develop customized drugs based on an individual's unique DNA and inform treatment options, among other things.

Chapter 4
Brain Computer Interfaces

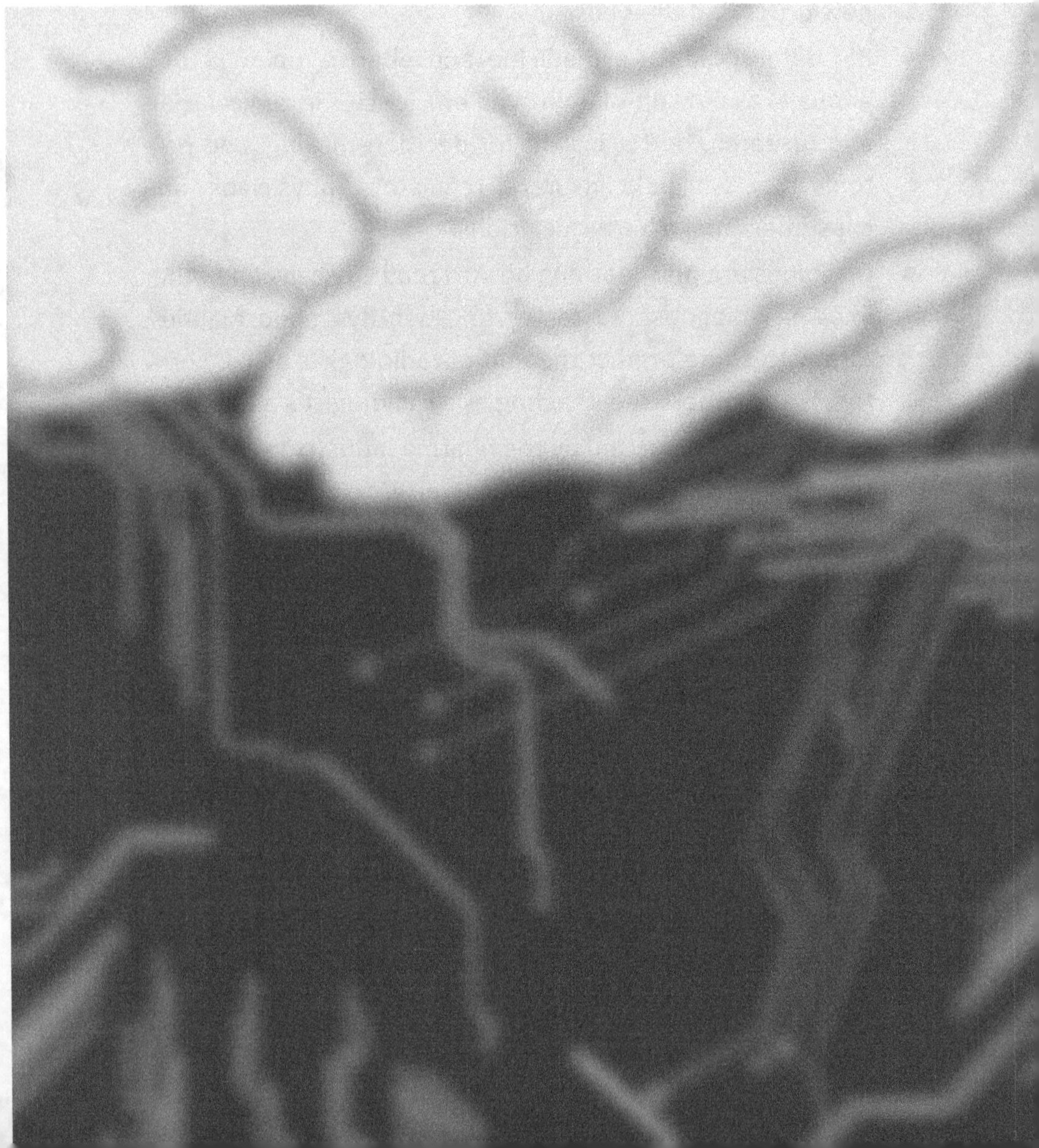

Contents

Introduction

It is part of human nature to invest in our curiosity and see where it leads. This curiosity has brought technological advancements that have revolutionized the healthcare and medical industries and will for centuries to come. However, in the search for a better comprehension of phenomena beyond our race, we forget that the most complex and least-understood network is within ourselves, the human brain.

Brain-computer interfaces (BCIs), sometimes called a neural-control interface (NCI), mind-machine interface (MMI), direct neural interface (DNI), or brain-machine interface (BMI), provide a direct communication pathway between an enhanced or wired brain and an external device. A BCI device measures the activity of the brain or central nervous system. It converts these signals into electronic signals to control and direct external devices, such as personal computers, robotic arms, wheelchairs, or activate a person's muscles. Some BCIs are combined with medical devices to increase communication or motor control for persons with physical impairments. BCIs have also been implemented in neurorehabilitation to improve neurological conditions such as motor paralysis after a stroke or spinal cord injury and epilepsy. Research has demonstrated many uses for BCIs, including medical benefits such as treating psychiatric conditions and neuro-enhancement to improve memory, increase mental alertness and concentration, and boost energy levels and wakefulness.

The innovation that kick-started BCIs was the electroencephalogram (EEG), invented by German Psychiatrist Hans Berger. This innovation was a breakthrough in neuroscience; it enabled human brain mapping and allowed brain activity to be recorded. While many physicians have used EEG since its invention in the 1920s, it wasn't until 1998 when neurologist Philip Kennedy implanted the first BCI into a human being, marking the day that the relationship between computers and humans changed forever. As time progressed, more technological advancements and BCIs were made and developed to an extent where they help scientists, physicians, and patients in endless applications. BCIs will serve as the path to further understanding of the human brain, improve and eliminate brain injuries and conditions, and increase human efficiency as a new technology that will revolutionize the healthcare industry.

What Is a Brain-Computer Interfaces?

Every human has a central nervous system (CNS). The CNS responds to stimuli, external or internal occurrences, by producing outputs specific to the stimulus. These outputs are generally in the form of muscular or hormonal actions, such as touch or feeling. However, in cases of paralysis or brain injury, often the CNS is too damaged to create such output. When treating patients with paralysis or brain injury, BCIs play an essential role. BCIs can reconnect the CNS to the rest of the body using a "bridge" to restore, replace, and improve CNS output to change the interactions between the brain's neural network and the internal and external environment.

BCIs analyze the acquired brain signals and translate them into commands executed by output devices (computers) to carry out the brain's desired actions. Medical companies, universities, researchers, and scientists have heavily invested in the research of BCIs because of their incredible range of applications. For example,

BCIs can replace and restore function to people disabled by neuromuscular disorders such as amyotrophic lateral sclerosis, cerebral palsy, stroke, or spinal cord injury by giving them the power to control computers through thought alone. Current research shows the many applications of BCIs in the healthcare industry potentially yield great medical benefits. These benefits range from treating psychiatric conditions, using neuro-enhancements to boost and increase memory power, increasing mental alertness and focus, to delivering an overall energy boost to the individual.

There are two major types of BCIs: non-invasive and invasive. Non-invasive BCIs record information from sensors placed on or very close to the skull. No surgery is required to implant the recording devices. The most common non-invasive BCI is the EEG. EEG-based BCIs monitor fluctuations, changes, and anomalies in cognitive states while the user does tasks in the workplace or at home. In contrast, Invasive BCIs are implanted under the skull directly into the brain using neurosurgery. Single unit BCIs detect the signal from a single area of brain cells, while multiunit BCIs detect multiple regions. In all BCI types, users receive real-time feedback on their brain activity output, most commonly through visual, auditory, tactile, vestibular, or proprioceptive (being able to walk or kick without looking at your feet feedback.) In addition, BCIs can also be passive or reactive. Passive BCIs monitor involuntary brain activity, such as mental workload or affective state. Reactive BCIs use brain activity changes resulting from an individual's voluntary focused attention on a specific external stimulus, primarily visual, auditory, or somatosensory (pressure, pain, or warmth). Active BCIs require the user to visualize an action, such as imagining moving a limb. Closed loop BCIs stimulate the brain with implanted electrodes by reading information from the brain rather than other parts of the nervous system. Many use this method in the treatment of epilepsy or psychiatric disorders.

Neurofeedback is the BCI technique that uses brain monitoring technology such as EEG. It's a method of teaching the brain to control an involuntary or unconscious bodily process to re-establish a severed (or non-existent) connection between the brain and the body's senses. Neurofeedback helps measure brain waves and provides feedback to teach the patient self-control of their brain functions using a feedback mechanism to retrain brainwave patterns. Scientists and physicians use neurofeedback to treat neurological conditions and disorders such as depression, autism, anxiety, sleep disorders, attention-deficit/hyperactivity disorder (ADHD), and schizophrenia. In 2020, a BCI program called FarmerKeeper was developed to maintain attention above a threshold to control a runner seeking lost farm animals. FarmerKeeper uses a consumer-grade BCI headset to read users' attention. Researchers designed FarmerKeeper to support neurofeedback therapies, emphasizing usability and user experience. During a 10-week deployment study, 26 children with severe autism used FarmerKeeper as a tool to help their condition. This study confirmed that all the children with autism showed improvements in their attention, attentional control, and sustained attention. The study also indicated that using BCIs to assist with neurofeedback therapies helped children gain control over specific areas of their brain to remediate behavioral changes and alleviate psychological suffering with the help of BCIs and neurofeedback.

Brain-Computer Interfaces Uses and Applications

Developers have optimized non-invasive BCIs to serve as one of the most revolutionary medical devices that have been put into use in the healthcare industry today. BCIs can help people with paralysis. Those who have any type of paralysis benefit when they use BCIs as neuroprostheses (devices that use electrodes to interface with the nervous system). The BCI acts as a bridge between the prosthetic and a patient's nerves that may have been damaged or may not function properly. BCIs allow paralyzed individuals and those with a neuromuscular disorder to use and control computer-based neuroprostheses by using brain activity alone, not through muscular movement. However, one of the biggest challenges most BCIs used for paralysis have is that it is invasive, and the benefits of BCI-aided treatments may not outweigh the risks of invasive neuro-implants.

Research indicates that BCIs for paralysis can be a part of the patients' everyday life, but it is essential to introduce them to the technology as early as possible. For example, early introduction after an injury gives the patient time to become accustomed to the technology and improve results quickly. A gradual transition from small non-invasive electrodes placed in the skull to an invasive technology can be more comforting for patients than making the transition all at once. A recent study surveyed 52 patients about their interest and possible use of BCI technologies with ataxia (a group of disorders that affect coordination, balance, and speech). Participants discussed their interests and attitude toward BCIs and showed a positive view toward BCI-aided treatment despite the invasive nature of the therapy as the benefits outweigh the risks.

Further studies will open the door for more effective treatment plans for patients suffering from ataxia, paralysis, and many other neurological disorders and diseases.

Less invasive methods for connecting an individual's brain with a computer are being developed. One of the biggest focuses of BCIs is to help patients regain control of their brain and repair damaged neural networks with the aid of computer-based neuroprostheses. The use of BCIs has led to extraordinary advancements in the healthcare industry. However, researchers continue to experiment with how effective the BCIs are in preventing health conditions at an early stage. With the added benefits of BCI technologies' connection to an individual's neural network and their cognitive awareness of their internal body, BCIs may partner with AI and machine learning systems to create a more compelling online healthcare platform. This effectiveness is precisely why researchers and scientists have started investigating applications of non-invasive BCIs that focus more on preventive medicine and cognitive enhancement rather than the treatment of diseases and disorders. Not only will non-invasive BCIs be easier to use and likely prove to be a more convenient implementation path, but wearable BCIs would also be less noticeable. This implementation would allow them to be more accessible to a larger group of individuals and amplify its preventive possibilities and treatment applications. BCIs will be seamlessly integrated into people's everyday lives and provide accessible, preventative, and easy-to-understand health care services.

Restoring the sense of touch is one area of treatment where BCIs excel. Researchers are developing BCI solutions that may imitate the feeling of touch in paralyzed patients. The solution consists of a robotic arm connected to the patient's brain through a BCI. This solution uses biomimetic mapping. Biomimetic mapping mimics a biologically inspired design of human-made processes, substances, devices, or systems that imitate nature. They use this to help capture the natural connection between cortical activity and a volitional arm or hand motion and then use this information to control a prosthetic arm or orthosis. The robotic arm provides sensory feedback based on the patterns recorded in the system transmitted from the electrodes implanted in the user's brain.

Speech recognition technologies are among the most widely adopted across many industries. There is a BCI solution that researchers have developed to help understand neural signals suitable for automatic speech recognition (ASR) to help people with speech impairments. Researchers investigate EEG, fMRI, MEG, and near-infrared spectroscopy as enabling technologies. Driving the new BCI tools is a rise in the prevalence of neurological disorders such as strokes and traumatic brain injuries, the emergence of brain-computer interface technology, and the increase in the adoption of BCI tools and services in healthcare. BCI research and development generates tremendous excitement in scientists, engineers, clinicians, and the general public. This excitement reflects the rich promise of BCIs, and eventually uses them regularly to replace or restore helpful function for people severely disabled by neuromuscular disorders; they may also improve rehabilitation for those who have strokes, head injuries, and other psychological conditions. Attributing to the expansion of the BCI health field is the increased application of BCI tools in drug discovery and delivery.

Apart from speech disabilities, restoring any of the five human senses, and serving as a neuroprosthetic, BCI technologies are mainly implemented and resorted to in times of risk in individuals and are used as a last resort for many diseases and disorders discussed. One of the most common and fatal medical incidences is seizures. Statistics from 2020 show that roughly 70 million people worldwide have epilepsy (recurring seizures). Although there have been advancements in epilepsy treatments, nearly 80% of people with epilepsy live in low- and middle-income countries. A study conducted in 2021 found that 30% of epileptic patients are resistant to drug therapy. So, while drug advancements may be effective for most individuals who have epilepsy, we must ensure we do not neglect the remaining 30%. The study exploited the potential of BCIs, and the closed-loop BCI predicted 45% of the seizures, whereas the remaining seizures were able to be detected. The closed-loop BCI will begin something extraordinary for BCI implementation for epileptic patients. The BCI used in this study was programmed to trigger simulation when a seizure is detected to abort the episode.

The BCI developed by this innovative group of scientists can only shorten the seizure duration. On the other hand, the BCI-aided treatment yielded a 72% decrease in seizure activity duration. The highlight of this team's BCI system is that it simultaneously focuses on prevention and treatment. The combined system better aligns with the opinions of patients, physicians, and the vast majority of the healthcare industry. This team of scientists aims to develop their BCI technology to abolish seizure activity in epileptic patients. Using this technology for patients suffering from epileptic shocks is the best way to use closed-loop BCIs in the future. Furthermore, in the future, BCIs will likely only be used as a last resort for individuals that require treatment unless there is the continued development of non-invasive applications of BCI technologies. Additionally, BCIs may transition into the daily lives of individuals who are perfectly healthy to ease human living. However, the goal of using BCIs in treatment is to achieve prevention. The use will be only when there is a need for treatment or a plan for prevention with BCI support.

Due to the invasive nature of current BCI implementation techniques, the most common people who use BCI treatments are patients participating in clinical trials or patients in need of neuroprostheses. For instance, patients suffering from neurological conditions, such as neurological disorders, would register for clinical trials. The clinical trial would revolve around BCI-aided prevention and treatment for the patients participating in the clinical trials. The patients in a clinical trial can benefit the participants and the individuals executing the clinical trials. The patients would receive constructive feedback from the participants and help adjust parameters or control variables in the BCI-aided treatment. Overall, this will yield better results in potential future clinical trials. Apart from that, individuals suffering from neurological disorders can be treated with BCIs to help them overcome deficits and regain order in their brain easier. These neurological diseases can range from ataxia to epilepsy, Bell's palsy, acute spinal cord injury, and the lists continue.

Apart from neurological diseases and disorders, one of the most common groups of individuals who use BCIs now and in the future are patients suffering from paralysis. Typically, paralysis is a loss of ability to move some or all of your body resulting from illness, poison, or injury. To regain control of one's neural pathways and move the paralyzed parts of their body again, paralysis patients can opt for BCI-aided treatments where BCIs would help the individual regain connection with their affected areas of the body.

The aid of BCIs would allow for neural feedback, thus leading to the possibility of moving the body part(s) once again.

An even more common group of individuals who use BCIs are amputee patients. The amputee patients can use neuro-prosthetics to replace their amputated body parts. They use a computer-based prosthetic, paired with a BCI, to regain the sensation of using their limbs again through artificial neural stimulation. This application of BCIs is the beginning of this developing technology, and future applications look limitless. Futuristic applications range from day-to-day tasks from social media interactions to helping military personnel. One example of future applications is the shift from Facebook's BCI initiative. Facebook is now opting out of invasive BCI implementations and is focusing on groundbreaking wearable BCIs that allow users to type and interact with social media apps by simply imagining themselves having a conversation or typing. These futuristic advancements appear exciting, but researching scientists will require extensive research and testing during the early stages of BCI technologies. In addition, it is essential to continuously monitor and assess any security risks involved with BCI usage, whether that be in social media applications, military applications, and in the healthcare industry and for medical conditions treatment.

As research makes progress into BCIs and a better understanding of the technology, the brain-computer interface is one of the most promising and increasingly popular technologies for assisting and improving communication/control for motor paralysis (e.g., paraplegia or quadriplegia) due to stroke, spinal cord injury, cerebral palsy, and amyotrophic lateral sclerosis (ALS). Due to the endless potential that BCI technologies possess as researchers continue to find various applications for BCIs, the significance that BCIs hold becomes substantially more evident. This significance reflects the medical applications in the healthcare industry, it reflects day-to-day usage and specific usage for government organizations and the milirary, and the list continues.

Today, the goal of BCIs is to replace or restore helpful function to patients suffering from neuromuscular diseases. An example of conditions BCIs can help with is amyotrophic lateral sclerosis, cerebral palsy, stroke, or spinal cord injury. BCI research has extended to the ability to repair damaged brain areas and provide new functionality for people with paralysis. One of the most advanced BCI in this area is the transcranial magnetic stimulation (TMS) implant. TMS is a method of delivering electrical stimulation to the brain at various frequencies or stimulus intensities. Physicians use this electric stimulation to relieve symptoms of major depression when standard treatment does not work. Physicians stimulate the nerve cells in the brain that are associated with mood regulation to help correct the imbalance. Researchers are looking into utilizing TMS for other psychiatric/neurologic disorders such as alcohol dependence, Alzheimer's disease, post-traumatic stress disorder (PTSD), panic disorder, obsessive-compulsive disorder, epilepsy, and migraines.

Reflecting on the technological advancements BCIs have made since the 1970s, the potential for progress in technology with BCIs is clear. That clear potential continuously drives research and pursuit of improvements in BCIs today in all parts of the world. Apart from the potential BCIs possess in present and futuristic present day applications, they also can serve as a path to enlightenment for scientists and researchers to give individuals a better understanding of the most complex and least-understood object in the universe, our brain. BCIs can lead to discoveries and breakthroughs in subconscious brain activities, lead to a better understanding of early childhood development, open up new branches in neurological studies, and can revolutionize humans' day-to-day practices on a scale that will be ever-expanding.

In addition to BCIs serving as a path to neurological discovery and enlightenment, it is also vital that the healthcare industries and other industries opt to use BCIs because they help patients, healthcare providers, and even individuals performing day-to-day tasks. For healthcare providers for the elderly or disabled individuals, BCI implementation can assist with domestic chores and remove communication barriers. This implementation will significantly enhance the patients' quality of life and relationships by strengthening their cognitive and motor abilities. The development and later usage of BCIs are essential because they will ensure that healthcare providers, the healthcare industries, and patients all experience a smooth and easy transition into using this technology.

The Future of Brain-Computer Interfaces

Outside of laboratories and experimental facilities, the most commonplace to find BCIs is in hospitals. Physicians will assist patients with BCI-aided treatment plans as a part of neurorehabilitation. One form of BCI is known as Hybrid Visual-BCI (V-BCI). It is used explicitly in hospital settings to grant patients control of prosthetic computer-based devices and assist them in their day-to-day tasks by overcoming the individual's barriers they may face due to a neurological disorder or disease. For patients with recent amputations due to an infectious disease or paralysis, nurses and physicians could implement the Hybrid V-BCI to assist their rehabilitation. The Hybrid V-BCI ensures that the patients have a smooth transition into their new way of living while always prioritizing the patient's comfort. The most common use of this technology in a hospital setting is when patients opt for a robotic prosthetic that is often paired with a BCI mechanism to ensure a successful link between the patient's brain and the robotic prosthetic. This BCI link allows the patient to interact with the neuro-prosthetic naturally and makes the transition more accessible and comfortable.

A close second to a hospital setting, another place to find the usage of BCIs would be in clinics where there are clinical trials. The primary purpose of clinical trials is to help researchers declare whether or not a new treatment plan or technology, in the case of BCIs, is safe and effective to use publicly or frequently as a treatment. Clinical trials are the most critical and respected stage of treatment development. Without successful results from a clinical trial, further implementation is not encouraged and is usually not pursued. For instance, an academic journal published in 2021 suggests that with the help of BCIs, it is possible to detect error correlation using motor-imagery-based BCIs. The motor imagery can help with error correction, prevention, and online updating or adjustment of the BCI in the motor cortex of an individual's brain. In other words, the clinical trial would aim to focus on error prevention for humans. If there are errors in the motor cortex, the BCI can detect the error, update, and correct those mistakes to prevent these errors in the future. This clinical trial has the potential for optimizing day-to-day human tasks and can make the lifestyle of many, if not all, individuals significantly more efficient.

These are just a few of the current whereabouts of BCIs in the present day. There is continuing research on BCIs for futuristic applications, including military usage. There are proposals for advancements in BCI that will eventually provide remarkable military advantages to countries that develop BCIs. These military advantages include heightened situational awareness, enhanced autonomous system management, human cognitive enhancement beyond natural abilities, synthetic telepathy, augmented reality/response, improved training techniques, and reduced casualty rates with improved medical outcomes. BCIs made for military applications can also be transferred to non-military settings such as a hospital environment or even day-to-day tasks that individuals do outside of their work life. These advancements in BCIs show the potential, and it will be remarkable to see where else they will be implemented soon.

With the quick advancement in technology today, it feels as though we are all heading toward becoming cyborgs, with computers running half of our day-to-day activities. We could check the news, screen our health, see what vitamins we need, track the physical fitness we perform, start our car and send an email to our boss, all without lifting a finger. Between the inserted invasive BCIs to the non-invasive wearable BCIs, the future of brain to computer technology is endless.

Risks and Challenges

BCIs are a relatively new and developing technology, which implies that apart from controlled settings, such as a hospital or clinical environment, it is unlikely that individuals have access to them. An additional reason for the lack of accessibility is the concern for the privacy and data security of the individual. When BCIs are not in a controlled setting, there can be complications familiar and unfamiliar to researchers. The release of BCI technologies for the public to use of their own volition does not currently have a date. The hesitancy is because there are very few wearable and non-invasive methods of implementing BCIs. Because of the lack of non-invasive techniques, it is strongly discouraged and advised against individuals to plant BCI technologies into their own body (brain) without the supervision of a professional in the field present. Even at that extreme, the technology is quite difficult to implant into oneself without causing any irreversible damage to themselves and their brains. Scientists always recommend that a professional, other than the individual seeking the BCI-aided treatment, execute the implementation processes.

An academic journal published in 2021 emphasizes the lack of reliability that Mental-Tasks-based Brain-Computer Interfaces (MT-BCI), a popular and commonly used BCI, have outside of a laboratory setting. The journal suggests that this challenge stems from humans using the technology rather than the technology itself. The article states MT-BCIs require their users to develop the ability to self-regulate specific brain signals. However, the human learning process to control a BCI is still relatively poorly understood and how to optimally train this ability is currently under investigation.

In the past, while initially developing BCI technologies, neuroscientists studying in the field of neuroethics began to take note of the complex nature of BCIs. They worried about the artificial implications of the therapies and whether or not they were effective. In an recent study about how living with a computer in their brain affects individuals, of the six individuals interviewed, all of them are comfortable with the BCI-based treatments. Some patients described the effects of the treatment as "radical symbiosis." The overall result was positive, with patients feeling a co-existence with their BCI. Furthermore, because of the increase in usage and the growing implementation of epilepsy treatments, the efficiency and reliability of the technology are increasing due to the constant feedback the BCI scientists and researchers receive from users. However, this raises the challenge of data security and patient confidentiality, for which skeptics still presume that giving computer access to the brain's neural pathways can lead to thought theft, neural corruption, and overall harm to the brain's organic health.

Beyond concerns with brain health, many security issues and problems revolve around this technology. They all stem from data privacy and the security of information retrieved from the brains of the individuals that use BCIs. Many researchers and BCI-focused companies are exploring whether BCIs can be used to read the thoughts and understand the neural processes of individuals. Scientists hypothesize that perhaps, sometime soon, BCIs will help neurologists understand one of the most mysterious parts of the human brain, and that is our subconscious. As this technology is further researched and developed over the years, companies and organizations intend to use this technology to revolutionize the way we interact without computer-based devices. A project launched by Facebook in 2017 focuses on using BCIs to grant users the ability to use a wearable device that will allow them to type by simply imagining themselves talking. Although, this wearable device approach from Facebook is their second approach. They first succeeded in decoding words through brain activity by implanting invasive nodes into a paralyzed patient who could not speak. The company decided, going forward, to opt out of invasive techniques with BCI, and is now focusing on wearable technologies. The challenge other companies like Facebook face now is the security of this technology. This worry stems from the user's data safety because, with a neural link that can connect thoughts to actions, it is hard for users to trust that their data is safe.

In addition, ethical complications such as data privacy and thought protection are some of the biggest challenges for BCI implementation. Neural information is some of the most private and intimate information. To put that in the hands of someone wanting to harm others could be disastrous. Researchers say that despite the positive progress so far, once BCIs are mature enough for various mind-reading tasks and used in multiple scenarios, it is nearly impossible for individuals to keep their thoughts private, which will lead to a great challenge for personal privacy and human agency.

Will employees be at the risk of their employers reading their minds? Could someone lose a job simply because of a fleeting thought? Furthermore, one of the additional potential downsides to implementing BCIs in the medical field and healthcare industry stems from the lack of accessibility of the technology. BCI implementation is an expensive and invasive medical treatment that only a select group of individuals can afford. The question is, is it fair that empowered people will benefit more than those who did not use that technology? Also essential to acknowledge the safety and health risks associated with non-invasive BCI implementation. Even the non-invasive BCI can potentially cause more damage than the intended good. There may be many advantages and benefits to various BCI implementations today, but the patients and practitioners must not disregard the challenges.

Summary

The emerging technology of brain-computer interfaces provides a clear communication pathway between an enhanced or wired brain and an external device. A BCI device measures the activity of the brain or central nervous system. It converts these signals into electronic signals to control and direct external devices, such as personal computers, robotic arms, wheelchairs, or activate a patient's muscles. BCIs aims to decode human intentions leading to direct brain control of a computer without needing to use the neuromuscular pathway. Either through invasive or non-invasive implementation strategies, BCIs can connect the brain's neural network to a computer-based system that converts neural signals into a tangible output. This conversion typically occurs through neural feedback; however, advancements in BCIs show that data storage can also aid in BCI-related functions. For instance, BCIs possess the potential to record error correlation with ensuring that the output does not repeat the detected mistake. This advancement in BCIs further emphasizes the potential of BCIs and how they can not only treat patients suffering from neurological conditions and paralysis but also pave the way for enlightenment in the field of neuroscience.

Through this enlightenment, researchers will continue looking into getting even more information about the human brain. Microscopic sensors that use ultrasound to record electrical signals from neurons are called neural dust (a term referring to millimeter-sized devices operated as wirelessly powered nerve sensors). So far, the research for neural dust is on the peripheral nervous system (the nerves that work throughout our limbs). Still, additional improvements could allow scientists to use the technology in the brain and central nervous system. If scientists recorded signals from sensors all over the body, they could have a complete view of neural activity and better understand how to harness and enhance it.

BCIs will also augment the performance of surgeons or other medical professionals. As neuroscience evolves and uses invasive and non-invasive technology alongside it, they will be able to view the brain, treat illness, and enhance cognition. Beyond treating conditions, BCIs are currently used to help treat paralysis and neurological disorders such as epilepsy and ataxia. Many fields see the benefit of BCIs, even the social media company, Facebook, is developing and researching BCI technologies to revolutionize the way individuals use and interact with social media. They are trying to develop wearable technologies that allow individuals to communicate and interact with social media platforms simply by thinking about them. Even government organizations, such as the military, see potential benefits regarding soldier health, field advantages, and analytical uses. Despite these advancements, it is essential to know that BCIs are here to help revolutionize the healthcare industry, optimize medical treatments for patients suffering from neurological disadvantages and increase convenience in the day-to-day lives of humans on an international scale. While technology will undoubtedly revolutionize the healthcare and medical industry, it is crucial to prioritize the safety and privacy of individuals, and until further research does not reassure the users of this, investigations and research must continue.

Statistics and Trends

- Brain-computer interface (BCI) technology is now being incorporated into treating many patients suffering from cognitive or physical impairments. This technology promises to significantly enhance these patients' quality of life by considerably improving their autonomy and mobility.
- BCI systems could be helpful for older adults in many ways, such as (1) training their motor/cognitive abilities to prevent the aging effects, (2) controlling home appliances, (3) communicating with others during daily activities, and (4) controlling an exoskeleton to enhance the strength of the body's joints.
- Brain-computer interface is one of the most promising and increasingly popular technologies for assisting and improving communication/control for motor paralysis (e.g., paraplegia or quadriplegia) due to stroke, spinal cord injury, cerebral palsy, and amyotrophic lateral sclerosis (ALS).
- In 2021, the BCI market was worth $185.21 million worldwide. The market is forecast to grow by 12.43% in the coming years, reaching a projected $393 million.
- Although the most common use of BCI is to help disabled people with disorders in the motor system, it might be a valuable tool for improving the quality of life of healthy people, particularly the elderly.
- Non-invasive BCIs have been used for restoring memory and planning using electromagnetic stimulation and biofeedback that modulate activity in a patient's brain as part of a rehabilitation program.

- One of the most significant challenges in BCI technology is the development of less invasive or non-invasive technologies for paralyzed patients. Using non-invasive devices can significantly reduce both the total cost of surgical operation and the physical harm to the patient.
- Brain imaging technologies such as Magnetoencephalography (MEG), functional Magnetic Resonance (fMRI), Electrocorticography (ECOG), and Electroencephalography (EEG) are integrated with BCI systems to capture electrical signals sent by the human brain.
- The segment's growth is attributed to the rise in the adoption of non-invasive brain-computer interface systems. These are used to control robotic arms, beneficial for paralyzed people.
- The invasive BCI segment is expected to witness the highest growth in the upcoming years as it is directed implanted in the brain and has the highest quality signals.
- Invasive BCIs are also used to restore vision by connecting the brain with external cameras and to restore the use of limbs by using brain-controlled robotic arms and legs. These benefits of invasive BCI are expected to fuel the demand in the upcoming years.
- The software segment is expected to witness the highest growth in the upcoming years as there has been an increase in the adoption of BCI software among the end-user, ensuring the effective functioning of BCI platforms.

Chapter 5
Nanomedicine

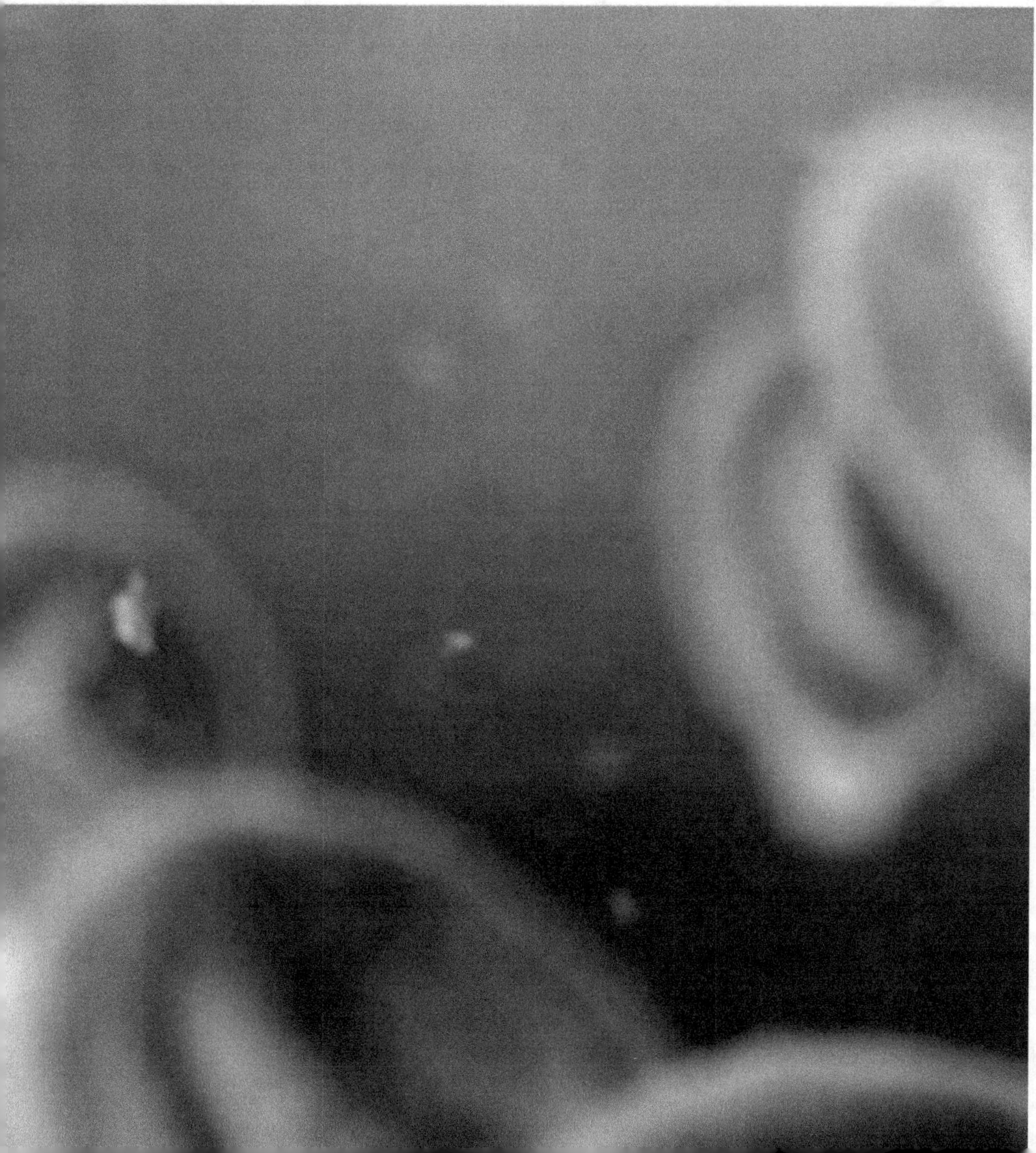

Contents

Introduction

The world's first computer was about 50 feet in length, weighing 5 tons, and now the smallest computer is less than the size of a grain of rice, measuring 0.3 mm in length. In this fast-pacing world, modern science is moving towards more compact, more precise, and more efficient technology, and medicine is no different. Nanomedicine is a revolutionary technology in the 21st century that has the potential for promising changes in healthcare leading to exciting medical breakthroughs.

Nanomedicine may be new to the world but not the technology per se. Its history can be traced back to the late 15th century when colloidal gold, also known as nanogold (a colloidal suspension of nanoparticles of gold in a fluid, usually water), was used to treat melancholy. The concept of nanotechnology was predicted by American Physicist and Nobel Prize winner Richard P Feynman in 1959, who even mentioned the scope of utilizing this technology in medicine. This opened the doors to new research fields in producing nanostructures and using them to diagnose and treat various diseases.

The evolution of nanomedicine as modern revolutionary science is possible only because of the development of ultramicroscopic devices, which led to a better understanding of molecular biology and physiology of various intra and intercellular processes. This remarkable progress in nanobiotechnology became the basis of nanomedicine. Today nanomedicine research and product development are used in imaging contrast agents, biomarker detection, nanotoxicology, and cancer treatments helping immune cells engage and subsequently eliminate cancer cells through target-oriented drug delivery.

What is Nanomedicine?

In simple terms, nanomedicine is the medical application of nanotechnology. Nanomedicine uses nano-sized tools for the diagnosis, prevention, and treatment of disease and to gain an increased understanding of the complex underlying pathophysiology of the disease. The ultimate goal is to improve the quality of life. To understand more about this, we need to know how small the nanoscale is. A nanometer is a unit of measurement that is equivalent to one-billionth of a meter or 0.000000001 meters. If we compare the nanoscale to objects, a human hair is about 60,000 – 100,000 nm wide, and a fingernail grows 1 nm per second.

In addition, nanomedicine is the application of nanotechnology to achieve innovation in healthcare. It uses the properties developed by a material at its nanometric scale, which often differs in physics, chemistry, or biology from the same material at a bigger scale. Moreover, the nanometric size is also the scale of many biological mechanisms in the human body. It allows nanoparticles and nanomaterials to potentially cross natural barriers to access new delivery sites and interact with DNA or small proteins at different levels in the blood or within organs, tissues or cells.

Nanomedicine has the potential to enable early detection and prevention and to drastically improve the diagnosis, treatment, and follow-up of many diseases, including cancer. Overall, nanomedicine has hundreds of products under clinical trials, covering all major conditions, including cardiovascular, neurodegenerative, and musculoskeletal. Enabling technologies in all healthcare areas, nanomedicine already accounts for approximately 80 marketed products, ranging from nano-delivery and pharmaceutical to medical imaging, diagnostics, and biomaterials.

Nanomedicine Uses and Applications

Nanomedicine can include a wide range of applications, including biosensors, tissue engineering, diagnostic devices, and many others. It involves harnessing nanotechnology to diagnose, treat, and prevent various diseases more effectively. Currently, nanomedicine technology is used in multiple diagnostic approaches such as ultrasound contrast agents, treatments of cancers like leukemia, iron deficiency anemia, AIDS, and age-related macular degeneration. It is also used in developing vaccines such as the Hepatitis A vaccine, Influenza vaccine, and the COVID19 vaccine.

A significant area of current use for nanomedicine is its ability to bind to biological molecules with extremely high specificity. Because nanoparticles can be engineered to have different sections attracted to specific cells, these nanoparticles can deliver other molecules to those exact sites. This process of precision locating allows medical professionals to use nanoparticles for a variety of uses. A nanoparticle may have an additional section that allows for imaging by being fluorescent or having a molecule that may interact with an imaging device. This enables physicians to precisely locate the type of tissue the nanoparticle is designed to bind to. Alternatively, the nanoparticle may have a section that can act as a treatment for the specific target tissue. This is often used in chemotherapy to treat cancer tissue that the nanoparticle can bind to. This precision treatment allows for safer and more controlled use of toxic pharmaceuticals. A patient may be able to undergo chemotherapy without serious side effects such as hair loss and stomach problems. The precision and ability for nanoparticles to transport molecules to a precise location inside an individual has been used for over 10 years now in clinical settings. It continues to be a point of research for the precision administration of specific molecules to specific locations within the body.

Another area of nanotechnology in medicine is the development of membranes that consist of nanoparticles or have nano-sized holes (nanopores) in them. These nanomaterials can be used for a wide range of medical processes such as drug delivery, where the material may encapsulate the drug; DNA sequencing, where a single DNA strand may be fed through a nanopore; and biocompatibility, where a nanomaterial may be used to enhance the regrowth of bone. These applications are various uses of the nanomaterial section of the field. The applications of these materials, which have specific and unique properties, not unlike nanoparticles, are another helpful way that nanotechnology has been applied to the medical field to enhance healthcare. These nanopore materials have also allowed for the application of nanofluidics (the study of the behavior, manipulation, and control of fluids that are confined to structures of nanometer typically 1–100 nm) to medical applications. The ability to rapidly test for specific select biological molecules that may signal disease, infection, or a deviation from homeostasis is essential for cost-effective early detection and emergency care. These minuscule and selective pores in materials allow medical professionals to note the presence of specific molecules without extensive or destructive testing.

Current research and innovation in nanotechnology are in applications in regenerative medicine and tissue engineering. Because nanoparticles and nanomaterials can be engineered to have structures, matrices, and lattices that mimic biological tissue, this can often improve many tissues' regenerative and growth capabilities. The introduction of a nanomaterial "scaffold" that allows for natural tissue to regrow has already been employed in bone, cartilage, nerves, cardiac tissue, and other tissues. The ability for these nanomaterials to interact with and absorb many biological molecules, including proteins needed for tissue regrowth, allows these materials to help regeneration when normal biologically produced healing processes are not sufficient.

The Future of Nanomedicine

The future is bright for nanomedicine. The field translates to a tremendous number of possibilities for expanding into multiple medical specialties and opening new prospects. Personalized medicine is the new vision of nanomedicine which, by techniques like molecular profiling (which identifies the unique DNA changes in a person's tumor), can deliver tailored individualized therapy. An increasing amount of research is being done in the direction of personalized nanomedicine because diseases such as cancer are highly heterogeneous, and the existing treatments are effective only for certain patients and patients at a certain stage of the disease. Through tailor-made medicines, it may become possible to develop effective and well-tolerated treatments for diseases that have so far been incurable.

Nanotheranostics is a multi-component system incorporating both diagnostic and therapeutic molecules in a single entity that allows for the diagnosis, drug delivery, and monitoring of the effects of the medicine by incorporating nanotechnology. It can be beneficial for even fatal diseases such as cancer, AIDS, and cardiovascular diseases by making the treatment less challenging and improving the prognosis, thus enhancing patients' quality of life.

Another exciting field of exploration is nano-based gene therapy, by which many genetic diseases which seem impossible to treat in today's time can be treated. This innovative technology in medicine stands to benefit from expanding the existing knowledge to more extensive clinical trials, adapting to technological advancements in healthcare, and working in a multidisciplinary approach to overcome challenges and barriers. Nano-based regenerative medicine combines nanotechnology with tissue engineering to create, repair, or replace tissues through targeted stimulation and growth, such as hair, skin, bone, nerve cells, muscles, or organs. This utilization of nanotechnology in regenerative medicine brings hope to treating incurable neurological diseases such as Alzheimer's, multiple sclerosis, and Parkinson's by targeted growth of nerve cells. If targeted manipulation of adult stem cells is also successful, endogenous tissue which is free of rejection reactions could be cultured, and embryonic stem cells could no longer be needed.

The technology could end drug resistance altogether, as the offending microorganisms would be targeted and disabled at a molecular level controlling many dreadful infectious diseases across the world. The future of nanomedicine will entail more advanced, more effective, and more cost-effective diagnostic systems and therapeutic devices that maximize positive outcomes and minimize the harm caused by the most devastating diseases we've ever encountered. With more and more researchers investing their time and energy into this groundbreaking technology, and many studies now entering clinical trials, we can expect some amazing breakthroughs in medicine soon.

Risks and Challenges

As is valid with any newly developed biotechnology, there is an inherent risk when implementing nanotechnology in clinical practice or procedure. While the large surface-to-volume ratio of nanoparticles enables a higher efficacy in applied therapeutic agents, it also increases the potential for adverse reactions within the body. This possibility of toxicity of nanoparticles meant to function as medical devices can lead to various disorders such as inflammation, immunoreactions, or cancer. Some negative reactions' exact causes and mechanisms are not entirely clear yet. Still, it is essential that any new sort of nanotechnology is tested and researched so that any potential side effects can be identified and addressed as needed for the safety of the potential patients and the environment.

Despite the potential for nanoparticles and nanotechnology to function as innovative means to administer medicine, it cannot be forgotten that, at least for the moment, nanoparticles will still be considered foreign substances by the human body. Certain types of carbon nanotubes, which are used in nanomedicine, act similarly to asbestos particles due to the nanoparticle's structure. This indicates that the implementation of such carbon nanotubes may lead to similar complications as asbestos exposure, causing lung damage. However, some positive findings also suggested that carbon nanotubes may not demonstrate short-term toxicity, which may help in its compatibility capabilities as nanotechnology evolves. Physical reactions to nanoparticles introduce the potential for other issues. If nanoparticles are not expelled from the body, they can act like any additional accumulation of foreign physical objects leading to complications at the site of buildup.

Studies have shown that nanoparticles can be toxic to the environment. However, a complete understanding of the risk assessment is needed. These preliminary studies illuminated the need for establishing a new discipline, nanotoxicology, to address the nano pollution by studying the detrimental effects of nanotechnology on the environment and biosphere. Another intriguing finding is the emergence of nanoparticles that make bacteria resistant to antibacterial drugs, which could be a sign that we should not ignore the long-term impacts of such tiny particles. Currently, the production and recycling of nanoparticles is a high energy-intensive process, which may cause further harm to the environment. To ensure sustainability and avoid unwanted consequences of this technology, intensive research is crucial, bridging the gap between rapid development and a better understanding of its toxic effects

Summary

Nanomedicine is a vital enabling instrument for personalized, targeted, and regenerative medicine by delivering the next level of new drugs, treatments, and implantable devices to clinicians and patients for real breakthroughs in healthcare. Beyond that, nanomedicine provides essential new tools to deal with the challenge of an aging population. It is thought to be instrumental for improved and cost-effective healthcare, one crucial factor for making medicines and treatments available and affordable to all

Mankind is still fighting against a high number of severe and complex illnesses like cancer, cardiovascular diseases, multiple sclerosis, Alzheimer's and Parkinson's disease, diabetes, as well as different kinds of serious inflammatory or infectious diseases like HIV. Most of these diseases have a tremendous negative impact on the patient himself and society and are linked to social and insurance systems. It is of utmost importance to face these conditions with appropriate means, primarily addressed by nanomedicine applications. Nanomedicine raises high expectations for millions of patients for better, more efficient, and affordable healthcare and has the potential to deliver promising solutions to many illnesses. From diagnosis to disease monitoring, going through surgery and chemotherapy or regenerative medicine, nanotechnologies virtually impact all fields of current medicine

Several areas of medical care are already benefiting from nanotechnology's advantages. The first nanotechnology-based targeted drug delivery systems are already on the market, and others are in clinical trials or, by far the most significant part, are under development. Another highly attractive area of nanomedicine is diagnostics at the nanoscale. The aim is to identify a disease at the earliest possible stage. Ideally, a single cell with ill behavior would be detected and cured or eliminated. New concepts for regenerative medicine give hope to many patients with organ failure or severe injuries. Today, artificial skin, bone, and cartilage are in an advanced stage of development and are partly already on the market.

It is of utmost importance to examine all possible side effects on human beings and the environment upfront with care and responsibility. Several global projects are already dealing with these fundamental issues. Also, ethical concerns and social acceptance have to be taken into account.

Statistics and Trends

- Areas of nanomedicine growth include drug delivery, biomaterials, active implants, diagnostic imaging, tissue regeneration, cardiovascular diseases, oncological diseases, neurological diseases, orthopedic diseases, infectious diseases, and others.
- The healthcare nanotechnology (nanomedicine) market was valued at $319.85 million in 2022, and it is expected to reach $4.46 billion by 2026.
- Increasing prevalence of chronic disease such as cardiovascular disorders, diabetes, and cancer are expected to boost demand for nanomedicines.
- Therapeutics segment is expected to account for largest revenue share in the global market for the development of nanoemulsions and nanoformulations to address issues related to non-specificity and cell membrane barriers.
- Dendrimers segment is expected to register significant revenue growth over the forecast period as the most effective drug delivery option due to their unique structure allowing for a controlled-release of the drug.
- Increasing concerns related to toxicity and environmental impact of nanomaterials and stringent regulatory approval procedures are expected to hamper market growth to a certain extent.

- Some potential applications of nanomaterials in healthcare include highly targeted delivery of genes and drugs, precise engineering and regeneration of bodily tissues, contrast enhancement for MRIs, enhanced detection of proteins and pathogens, fluorescent labeling and tagging of proteins.
- Cardiology is anticipated to exhibit the fastest progress owing to the presence of opportunities such as demand for specific therapeutic nanovectors, nanostructured stents, and implants for tissue regeneration.
- Healthcare companies are targeting the treatment of several cancer types and infectious diseases through immunotherapy, where nanoemulsion vaccines and drugs play a significant role.
- In 2021, the FDA received 95 submissions for drugs containing nanomaterials.
- Carbon nanotubes can have a mechanical tensile strength 400 times greater than regular steel.
- Nearly 40% of humans will be diagnosed with cancer at some point in their lifetime. One of the key issues with conventional chemotherapy and radiation treatments is that the body's healthy cells can become damaged. For this reason, researchers around the world are working on using nanoparticles to specifically target cancer cells.
- Nanoparticles are able to give medical imaging techniques a clearer resolution, making it easier to identify the disease.
- Over the years, many nanomedicines have received clinical approval based on improved safety with equivalent efficacy.
- 32% of nanotechnology research comes from the U.S.

Chapter 6
Virtual and Augumented Reality

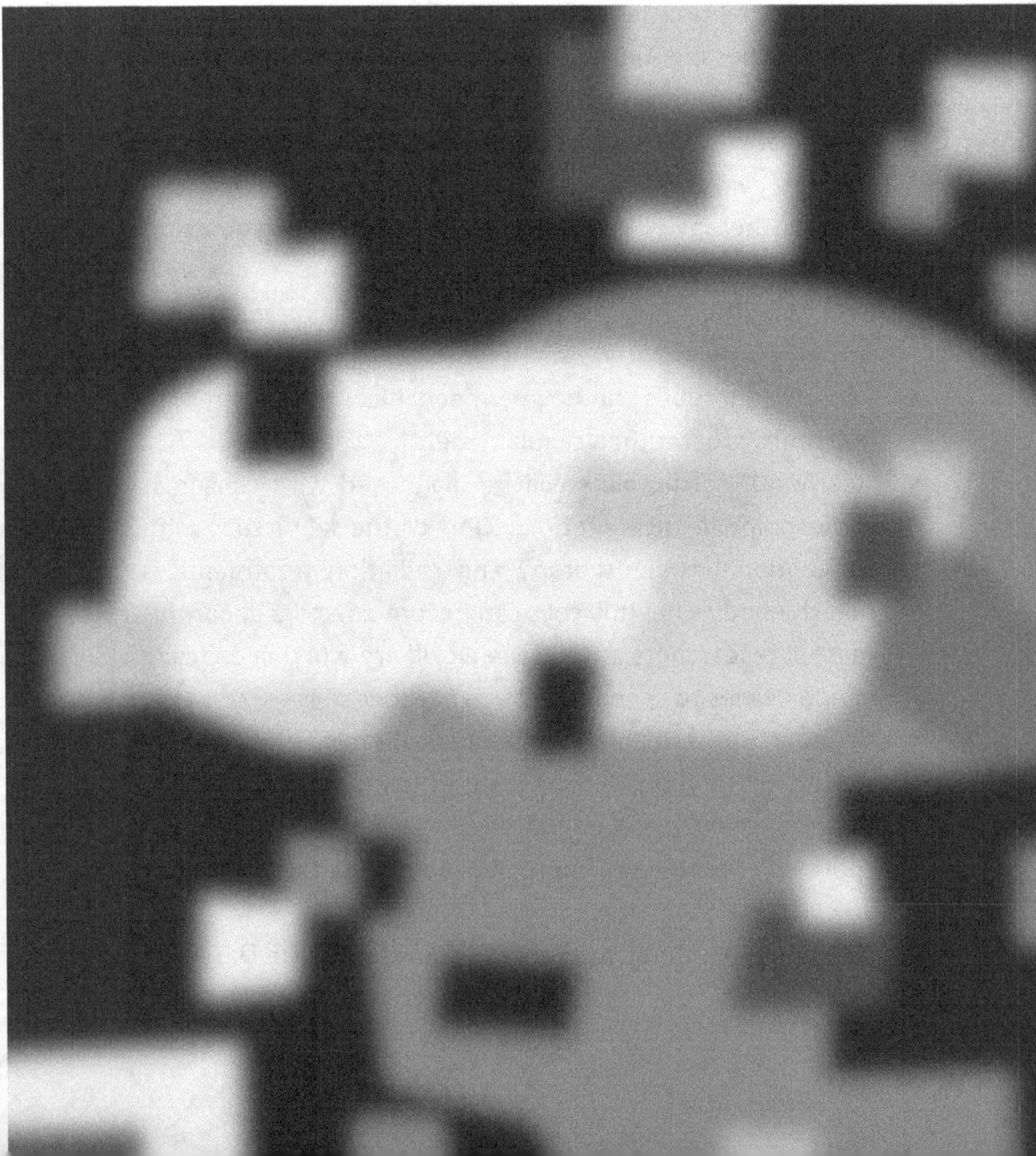

Contents

Introduction

In the last few years, virtual reality (VR) and augmented reality (AR) have become essential tools with various applications within the healthcare industry. VR is a technology that utilizes some type of head-mounted display to immerse the user into a 3D virtual environment completely. With the development of human-computer interfaces, VR users can see and interact directly with the digital world around them. Conversely, AR allows individuals to remain connected to the real world as they utilize it. AR technology includes 3D holograms and virtual environments displayed on a screen. VR and AR provide unique contributions to multiple aspects of the healthcare industry. VR can be utilized to improve surgical training within medical education, while AR can improve anatomy visualization.

Additionally, VR is an effective treatment for rehabilitation, mental health, and other psychological conditions. Not only that, but VR can also improve the quality of digital healthcare and online consultations. During surgical operations, AR can increase the precision of the procedure while also acting as a pain management tool for patients. In today's healthcare industry, there is a clear need to improve the quality and precision of medical practices. VR and AR are the best tools to deliver these advancements and replace outdated methods that are no longer beneficial to medical practitioners and patients. The following chapter will examine the various uses of VR and AR in healthcare, discuss the implications of this technology on the future of healthcare, and address the challenges that need to be overcome.

What is Virtual Reality and Augmented Reality?

On a fundamental level, VR technology creates a 360-degree virtual experience for patients through a 3D movie or panorama. The graphics are shown through a head-mounted display (HMD), which is a goggle-like device that completely covers the individual's visual field. VR HMD's can be either wireless or attached to a computer. Although the main focus of VR technology is the manipulation of the visual sense, recent developments have incorporated several more senses into the VR experience. For instance, multisensory devices can generate olfactory, tactile, and auditory feedback to individuals. VR typically utilizes hand-worn controllers to receive user input, such as joysticks and other consoles. However, these controllers are slowly being replaced by or combined with haptic (technology that stimulates the senses of touch and motion, especially to reproduce in remote operation or computer simulation) devices. Haptic technology adds a sense of touch to VR, allowing direct interaction with the virtual environment. Currently, haptic technology requires physical pressure sensors to give and receive tactile feedback, but future developments will enable touch sensitivity through vibrations and other advanced technology. New advancements in VR continue to be developed quickly, but the current technology is already very sophisticated and has countless applications within healthcare.

Conversely, AR does not completely immerse the user into the virtual world. Instead, it integrates virtual reality into the physical environment, making it a powerful tool within healthcare. Many different technologies are categorized as AR, the simplest of which include handheld devices and desktop applications. In these technologies, 3D graphics are shown on a 2D display. A more advanced and vital application would be a 3D model that projects the virtual content directly onto the natural environment, merging the two worlds using holographic technology.

Additionally, HMD-based AR systems superimpose virtual objects onto the physical environment through the goggle lenses, allowing the user to remain aware of the real world. AR can also contain interactive components where the movements of people and virtual objects are taken into account. Through this, AR can provide direct feedback to users and enhance the user's experience. Additionally, a subcategory of AR has triggered AR technologies, which activate based on a specific stimulus. For instance, location-based AR will start augmentation if the user visits a location point. AR has a unique flexibility that allows for broader implementations across the healthcare industry, from mobile apps to realistic holograms.

VR and AR Uses and Applications

Currently, one of the primary applications of VR technology is within medical training. Using VR, students can complete procedures, refine their skills, and take examinations without the constant guidance of an instructor. Within some fields, particularly orthopedic surgery, physicians cannot gain the necessary skills during their residency due to rising costs and availability. VR resolves this problem by eliminating the need for human and animal test subjects while also preventing the risk associated with resident physicians performing life and death procedures on patients. According to studies on a MIST-VR simulator, physicians trained using VR performed operations more effectively and caused fewer injuries than those who underwent traditional training. In addition to surgical training, VR is also integrated into dental education through Computerized Dental Simulators. Because of this training system, dental students can receive real-time feedback that is much more precise than the original, non-virtual training. Meanwhile, teachers can observe students and receive reports on their work while allowing students to engage in self-learning through VR. Thus, not only does VR prove to be a better learning tool for students, but it is also more efficient in saving teachers' time.

VR also has direct applications for patient treatment. For individuals with Parkinson's disease, VR rehabilitation treatment for their motor skills is more effective than traditional physical therapy. These results lie in VR's ability to provide automatic visual feedback for patients' posture and gait. Additionally, creative VR environments, including simulated travel and games, can improve patients' moods and decrease symptoms of depression. The most significant benefit of VR-based therapy is lifting the burden on caregivers since VR can significantly aid or eventually replace one-to-one physical therapy. Next, VR has applications for people with numerous psychological conditions, including PTSD, schizophrenia, phobias, and other mental illnesses. During PTSD diagnoses, patients' physiological reactions to virtual stimuli are analyzed to confirm their condition. After diagnosis, VR can also be utilized for PTSD treatment. A project launched in 2012 called Stress Resilience in Virtual Environments (STRIVE) taught stress reduction and emotional resilience that was particularly relevant to PTSD patients. Using VR, STRIVE created a narrative-based training that exposes patients to emotionally triggering events and then guides them through exercises to teach coping strategies. The results of the STRIVE project were positive, indicating VR's potential in therapy and treatment. This same model can be applied to patients with phobias through exposure therapy, especially given VR's ability to create highly immersive and realistic environments.

Another application of VR is its use as a distractor for patients. Research showed that 80% of VR headsets patients experienced less pain during surgery. VR can be an effective pain management treatment using cognitive behavioral therapy techniques. Moreover, VR can prevent cognitive deterioration in the elderly by providing psychological stimulation. VR may also become a treatment for dementia (a condition that impairs brain functions), but further research is required in this field. Lastly, VR can improve virtual health consultations by making them more interactive and personal than regular communication through a screen. To elaborate, VR can allow the patient to better understand their health by showing them interactive virtual models of their organs and physical condition.

Since AR allows the physician to remain connected to the real world while accessing the virtual world, it has practical applications during surgical operations. By integrating data from a CT or MRI scan into the AR system, the technology can provide navigational assistance or create a 3D visualization of the anatomy. An optical see-through (OST) display, which displays a semi-transparent graphic on the physical environment, can be used. Additionally, AR can allow physicians to conduct preoperative planning and surgery in a virtual environment before operating on the patient. This has been shown to significantly increase stability and precision during the operation, improving the success of life-saving procedures. Another form of AR is displayed on mobile devices, allowing life-saving technology such as defibrillator locators to be easily portable. For instance, AED4EU is an app that can project the location of defibrillators (a device that creates an electric current to restore a heart's beating) using AR, making them easy to find during crucial situations. It is also important to note that some VR health technologies have overlapping applications with AR. For instance, AR technologies are also utilized in pain management and medical education. However, AR's unique characteristics make it extremely important in the healthcare landscape alongside VR.

From the earliest development of head-mounted displays in 1965 to today, VR technology has undergone drastic changes. Ivan Sutherland first proposed the concept of an artificial world created with interactive graphics in 1965, marking the birth of VR. After a few decades, the VR field underwent essential developments, and the amount of VR research increased exponentially. During the late 1990s to the early 2000s, VR began expanding to multiple industries, including medicine. By 2016, large corporations started the widespread commercialization of VR, which kicked off a new era for VR. Today, many medical facilities and educational institutions utilize VR technology, and this number is expected to increase.

Although VR helps assist nurses, physicians, and surgeons, much of the existing research suggests that its most significant application currently lies within medical training. For instance, surgical training tools, such as the Virtual Surgeon, are already integrated into some medical education programs. However, given the speed of VR's development, it is inevitable that VR technology will quickly become more widespread across the healthcare industry. By 2025, the VR market size within healthcare will be worth 5.1 billion dollars, making it the third-largest industry utilizing VR. Within the next 20 years, head-mounted displays will be replaced by retinal scanning displays that can directly project graphics onto the eye. After the COVID-19 pandemic, virtual health consultations have increased 38 times after their initial peak. As the telemedicine industry grows, VR has more potential to be utilized more frequently within digital consultations by allowing patients to understand their conditions visually.

Additionally, by 2050, the elderly population will reach 2.1 billion, 46% of whom will be diagnosed with a disability. Thus, the burden on elderly caregivers will significantly increase, which creates a need for independent treatment technology, such as VR. As both the need for VR and its technological developments increase, the number of applications of VR in healthcare will continue to rise.

The development of AR did not begin until decades after Sutherland's first visualization of VR in the 1960s. When AR systems were developed to enhance fighter pilots' vision in the early 1990s, this new virtual technology began to take shape. By 2000, AR was being utilized for medical purposes. In comparison to VR, there is currently more literature on the clinical applications of AR, such as for surgery and rehabilitation. The majority of AR technology today focuses on visual augmentation, but future research will continue expanding on the augmentation of other senses. Likewise, past market trends show that the AR industry will only continue growing. AR will become increasingly available within the near future, allowing patients to have access to self-treatment. Thus, new forms of utilizing AR will be continually developed to improve healthcare services.

Although it is relatively simple to purchase VR video games, VR health technologies are not as readily available. That being said, there are still many biotechnology companies developing VR products. This includes FundamentalVR, a company that focuses on virtual surgical training, and OxfordVR, which develops VR for mental health disorders and phobias. However, it is challenging to find VR technology in rural areas and low to middle-income countries (LMICs), which may benefit the most from using it. In the past, it was unfeasible to provide emergency medical simulation training to LMICs because of the high cost that the machines required. Given VR's advancements that have made it less costly, it is the perfect tool to assist LMICs. In 2019, Oxford University introduced VR training to healthcare education in Kenya. After some time, the VR training improved their clinical skills significantly. Thus, VR has the potential to transform healthcare systems in many LMICs. On another note, VR is also an essential tool in the shift to at-home and digital healthcare. With VR equipment, patients can have treatments in the comfort of their homes.

Additionally, VR can be used to improve remote health consultations. With VR, feedback from the physician can be given in a great variety of ways. The physician may also monitor the patient's condition more clearly than with current and former telemedicine techniques. They can also explain the patient's medical condition more clearly with the help of virtual anatomy models. Thus, the healthcare setting can dramatically shift to maximize the comfort of patients

The diversity of AR health technologies indicates the variety of healthcare manufacturers involved in their creation. First of all, many AR technologies can easily be found within a smartphone's app store. However, even though there are numerous free apps available, some of the applications require purchasing other equipment. Additionally, many companies and educational institutions also focus on developing advanced AR health technology. For instance, Augmedis and Medivis focus on aiding physicians during surgical operations through real-time guidance and displaying the patient's anatomy before the surgery. SentiAR develops technology that can create a hologram of a patient's organs. At the same time, Medical Augmented Intelligence uses AR to train physicians in anatomy and even acupuncture. The countries leading AR development are the U.S., the United Kingdom, and China. Given its potential within healthcare, many dedicated individuals are consistently working to improve AR technology and make it more accessible to physicians and patients.

The Future of VR and AR

Although some VR technologies can be relatively inexpensive compared to other advanced products, VR has not become widespread across the healthcare industry yet. However, the educational implementations of VR are increasing as many medical schools across the U.S. have begun to use VR in their curriculum. For instance, Stanford's School of Medicine teaches students about the brain's anatomy using VR technology to create a 3D realistic brain model. Stanford's head of neurosurgery uses VR as a rehearsal for his operations on patients. Other institutions utilizing VR educationally include Case Western University and the University of Michigan, which use VR to train physicians' communication skills.

Additionally, VR is slowly becoming adopted as a standard pain management tool. In 2015, Stanford Children's Hospital launched the Childhood Anxiety Reduction through Innovation and Technology (CHARIOT) program, which utilized VR to help children cope with pain during surgical procedures. However, VR does not seem to be as actively used in patient treatment outside of pain management. Given the large amount of research showing VR's effectiveness in therapy, rehabilitation, and more, it would be beneficial for patients to integrate VR into their treatments. In particular, VR would enable elderly patients to avoid cognitive deterioration through simulation training. However, it is important to note that VR is currently not widely utilized by hospitals in rural areas and educational institutions that receive little funding. Thus, increasing access to VR technology should be a priority for the healthcare industry. If these changes are made, VR technology has the potential to be available to all who may benefit from it.

The availability of AR technology is similar to VR, albeit with few significant differences. Unlike VR, some AR technologies are in the form of mobile apps, making them easily accessible to all. Currently, there are already a few free AR health apps that aim to improve the fitness and well-being of their users. FitAbs is one such app that uses AR to teach fitness exercises. Another app, Healium AR, displays a bright ball through the device's camera function, which helps with patients' meditation practice. Apart from mobile apps, many educational institutions also use AR within medical education, similar to VR. The University of California Irvine School of Medicine uses AR technology to project a hologram onto a mannequin to make the training simulation more realistic. Unlike VR, AR technology allows students to continue interacting with each other, which increases collaboration.

Additionally, Stanford's CHARIOT program utilizes AR for young patients to play virtual games or watch movies to distract from surgical procedures. AR allows patients to remain conscious of their surroundings, which may be necessary depending on the operation. Looking forward, advanced AR technology must become more readily available to all physicians, patients, and medical schools to improve the healthcare industry.

VR is an important technology that has the power to change many aspects of the healthcare industry. First, VR can be used in place of surgical procedures depending on the medical condition. A research study showed that VR treatment proved to be more effective than surgery when treating intermittent exotropia, a condition that causes the eye to turn inwards. Because surgery can be invasive, costly, and risky, it is vital to turn to alternatives such as VR whenever possible. Often, the quality of treatment will also improve when using VR. VR simulations that treat psychological conditions also produce favorable results compared to traditional therapy, according to a meta-analysis of 22 studies. Through VR's advantageous uses within medical education, the quality of physicians is also increased. Compared to traditionally taught surgeons, who often train with mannequins due to lack of availability and experience, VR-trained surgeons are exposed to more realistic scenarios and perform at higher rates. At the same time, VR also promotes self-learning, which decreases faculty costs. Additionally, VR solves the ethical concerns surrounding the use of animal and human test subjects during medical education, given the unlimited supply of virtual patients. By replacing invasive treatments, increasing healthcare quality, and addressing ethical concerns, VR will lead the future of health technology to create a better healthcare system.

Additionally, AR technology provides many essential assets to the healthcare industry. First, with the rise of AR mobile apps and low-cost AR equipment, AR has the potential to be both highly accessible and of low cost. In this way, AR technology can be used to direct patients to treat themselves if a physician is not available making healthcare accessible to more people. AR's ability to integrate the virtual world into reality makes it a powerful tool for physicians. The added precision that AR provides may make the difference between saving a life and making a fatal mistake during surgery. Because both VR and AR are effective pain management treatments, they may be able to replace pain medication drugs in some situations. Because of the possible consequences of using painkilling drugs, including health issues and potential addiction, using AR as a pain management tool will positively impact healthcare. Thus, physicians need to continue employing AR technology for the benefit of patients.

Risks and Challenges

The introduction of new technology always necessitates a consideration of the possible challenges involved. First, patients who undergo VR treatment may be put at risk for adverse side effects, such as cybersickness (nausea and vomiting) and aftereffects (disturbed motor skills and fatigue). In one study, 17% of neurological patients experienced side effects after using a VR treatment. Thus, the effects of VR technology need to be extensively tested and improved to ensure the safety of patients. Additionally, VR may also cause virtual escapism, where patients use VR to escape from their physical environment. For example, if VR allows disabled patients to experience free mobility, they may become addicted to using VR. In such scenarios, VR would be highly detrimental to patients by preventing them from accepting their physical condition and even causing them to lose touch with reality. Next, VR may also negatively affect the interpersonal connection between patient and physician. Instead of interacting directly with their patients, therapists may choose to use VR technology completely. This may be damaging because the relationship between a therapist and their patient is often necessary for the patient to trust the treatment and improve their condition. To address this potential issue, physicians should continue to directly communicate with the patient even while using VR treatment. For instance, they can guide the patient through the VR treatment using a speaker or converse with them before and after the experience. Given the importance of interpersonal interaction, VR is not likely to replace human healthcare workers. Rather, VR should be used to increase efficiency and availability within the healthcare industry. Lastly, VR's increased use for self-diagnosis, treatment, and learning raises the question of how much individuals should rely on VR. For instance, can medical students trust VR to teach them the correct skills accurately without direct instruction from a teacher? Can patients completely trust VR technology to accurately diagnose and treat them? If so, should they still approach a physician for additional help? All of these questions and concerns are extremely valid and should be addressed before the use of VR becomes widespread within healthcare.

With AR, some of the ethical concerns related to VR, such as side effects and escapism, are not as severe since the user remains connected to the real world. However, AR technology may still lead patients to confuse the augmented world with reality and withdraw from real-world interactions. Because AR is more realistic than television and other digital media, this technology may worsen the disconnection with reality that individuals face due to an increasingly digitized world. This effect is particularly significant within children who use AR treatment since they have not developed a strong understanding of the physical world yet. Additionally, although virtual and augmented technology has the potential to be easily accessible by cutting costs, it is likely that this advanced technology will be first utilized only by institutions that can afford to replace old methods. In fact, excluding a few research studies, most VR and AR technologies are only available in well-supported universities and hospitals. If action isn't taken to distribute VR and AR more widely to disadvantaged areas, the potential exists to exacerbate the digital divide. Finally, the consequences of bugs or malfunctions are extremely severe, especially given AR's application in aiding surgery. If the technology isn't tested to be certain of functionality, it would not be ethical to utilize it on patients.

Summary

This chapter began by introducing the potential of VR and AR technology to dramatically improve the healthcare industry by directly aiding physicians, caregivers, and patients. Current research has made a compelling case that VR and AR can be integrated seamlessly into hospitals and homes to increase the quality and precision of treatment. In particular, VR can be utilized for rehabilitation and mental health treatment, decreasing the burden of caregivers and therapists. As the elderly population grows, VR can fill the gap between the medical needs of the elderly and the number of caregivers available. In this way, VR will contribute to the shift from healthcare to homecare as self-treatment using virtual technology becomes increasingly available. Although the majority of VR and AR technology is centered on treatment after diagnosis, it can also be used for wellness and prevention. For instance, there are applications of VR that prevent cognitive deterioration and strengthen emotional resilience to minimize the risk of potential health issues. Additionally, the immersive nature of VR and AR technology makes them powerful pain management tools that are already being utilized by children's hospitals. Thus, VR and AR treatment can greatly improve healthcare practices and benefit patients.

Since VR can create highly realistic training simulations, its applications within medical education are significant. As this virtual technology becomes more widespread throughout medical schools around the world, a new generation of highly skilled physicians will be created. Furthermore, AR can create 3D visualizations that guide doctors while performing surgery. VR can be used during virtual health consultations and to enable physicians to collaborate remotely, reducing the geographic boundaries in healthcare. Overall, one of the most important characteristics of VR and AR technology is their increasing efficiency that has lowered costs significantly. Individuals can even access AR health technology for free on their mobile phones. Given their inexpensive nature, VR and AR also have the power to change the accessibility of healthcare technology. For instance, they can be introduced in rural and developing countries to improve their healthcare systems with minimal cost. As the healthcare industry realizes the potential that VR and AR hold, physicians and healthcare providers need to begin integrating more of this technology into current medical practices. With VR and AR, the healthcare industry will be able to truly progress forward and best fulfill the needs of patients.

Statistics and Trends

- Healthcare workers have to learn a considerable amount of information about anatomy and how the body functions. AR applications allow learners to visualize and interact with three-dimensional representations of bodies. It's also proving useful for patient education, allowing medical professionals to help patients understand surgical procedures and the way medicines work.
- Today, surgeons use several techniques to visualize the area they are to operate. Still, AR, which can project three-dimensional representations of the patient's anatomy into the surgeon's field of view, is likely to improve accuracy and outcomes for patients.
- The global healthcare augmented reality & virtual reality market is further segmented by application into surgery, fitness management, patient care management, pharmacy management, medical training & education, etc.
- The market for AR in healthcare is expected to reach $2.4 billion by 2026 including pain management, memory care, and medical training, among other things.
- The global VR and virtual reality in healthcare market size was valued at $2.4 billion in 2022 and is expected to reach $9.5 billion by 2028. The market is expected to expand at a rate of 27.2% from 2022 to 2028.
- In 2022, the market will witness an increase of 85% from 2020, owing to the shift in trends towards AR and VR applications and adoption in the healthcare sector.
- The global healthcare augmented reality & virtual reality market is segmented by end-user into hospitals & other

medical facilities, research organizations & pharmaceutical companies, diagnostics laboratories, and others.

- Devices such as head-mounted displays, smart glasses, and 3D sensors hold significant shares in the market for AR & VR in healthcare.
- AccuVein, which is in use in hospitals today, can project a map of a patient's veins onto their skin, making it easier for healthcare workers to find the vein the first time.
- Healthcare consumers already have had exposure to AR and VR. Some experiences include the ability to "try on" glasses via retailers' websites. Some companies offer similar solutions in the aesthetic medicine and orthodontia markets to give users a sense of the intended progress or result of a procedure.
- As patients remain isolated, healthcare organizations might consider launching or increasing VR programs for self-guided rehabilitation exercises and addressing chronic pain.
- VR and AR technologies are being used in operating rooms and classrooms to help surgeons prepare for the jobs ahead. Surgeons using AR and VR can walk through the organs they are about to operate on. This is profoundly changing the way surgeries are performed today.
- Instead of showing an X-ray to a patient and telling them what you're going to do, physicians can show them a 3D model of what will happen during the surgery and what it will look like afterward.

Chapter 7

Robotics and Robot Assisted Surgery

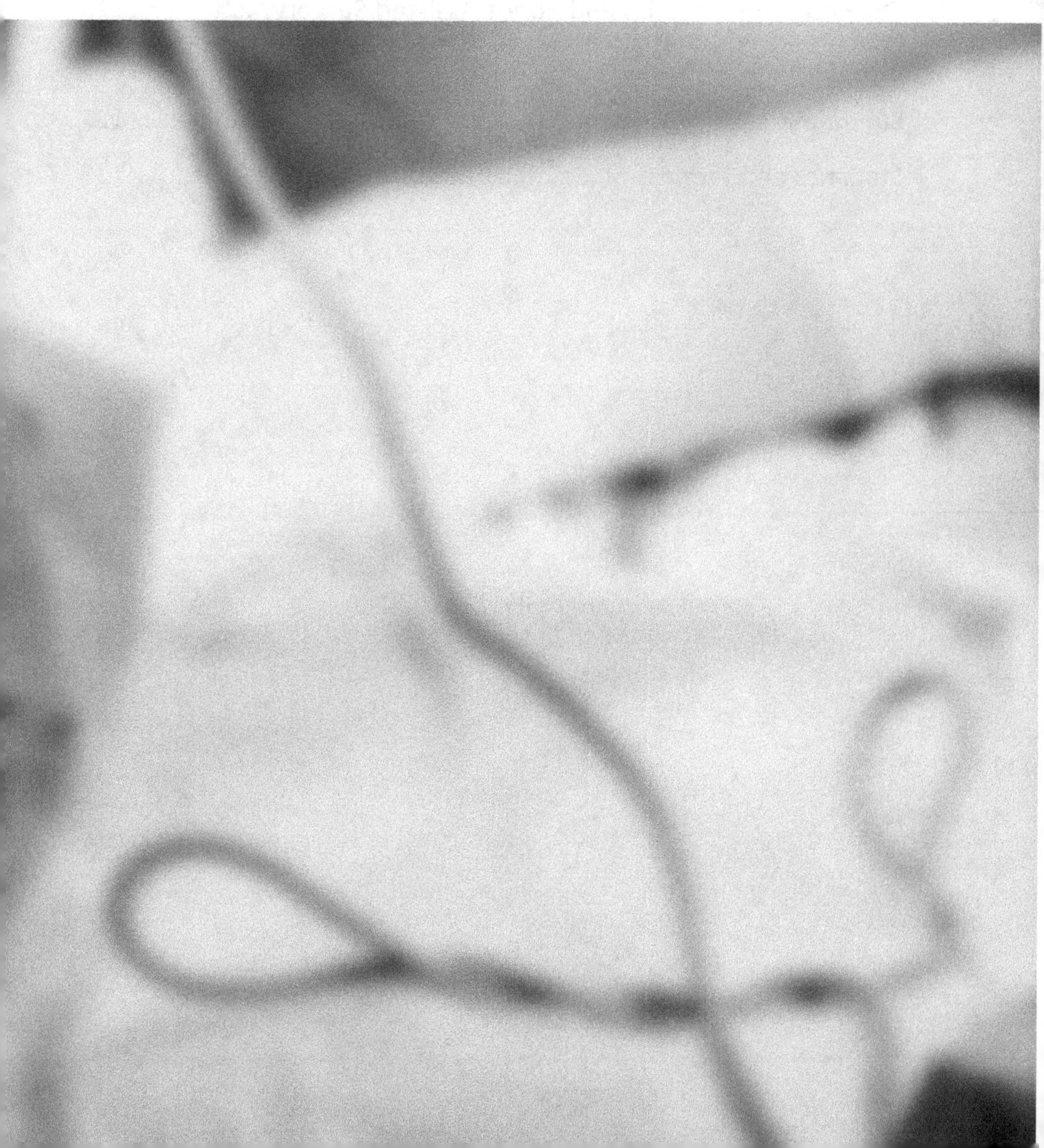

Contents

Introduction

With the technological advancements over the past few decades, it is no surprise that robots have become increasingly intelligent, autonomous, and valuable. Robotics is a computer science and engineering field where machines perform tasks initially done by humans. In some cases, robots can complete functions unachievable by humans or perform tasks better than even the most skilled professional. There is a large diversity of robot types that can do various activities and have varying levels of autonomy.

One of the largest and most important uses of robotics in healthcare is robot-assisted surgery. A surgeon uses controls to manipulate robotic surgical instruments, increasing the precision and quality of complex surgical procedures. Other uses of robotics in healthcare include robot companions, exoskeletons, microrobots, and others. Robots can also directly assist physicians and nurses. Given the increase in elderly patients, robot companions are crucial to supporting overworked caregivers. Robots can also make up for potential shortages of medical staff.

Additionally, robots can lead to greater accessibility of healthcare by revolutionizing telesurgery. Robotics provides many essential benefits that will positively change the healthcare industry with these applications. This chapter will describe the applications of robotics in healthcare and discuss the technology's impact on the medical field.

What is Robotics and Robot-Assisted Surgery?

Robotics is a technology field where machines complete tasks done initially by healthcare workers. Generally, the components of a healthcare robot include sensors, a computer system, and an output action. Sensors detect the patient's movement, speech, or other stimuli using 3D cameras, motion detectors, or speech recognition. The computer will then process the information from the sensors using AI systems like computer vision and other advanced processing models. Then, the robot will be programmed by the computer to perform an output, which can be in the form of a physical movement, speech, or any other action. Robots are classified as active if they can move independently from an operator under the influence of a computer program. On the other hand, semi-active robots are controlled by a physician, and their movements mirror those of the physician.

One of the most important and well-developed categories of healthcare robotics is robot-assisted surgery. Under a physician's control, the robot can make precise incisions and perform parts of the operation. A surgical robot typically consists of a remote control, robotic arms, surgical instruments, and cameras. Such robots can be classified as computer-aided design/computer-aided manufacturing (CAD/CAM) systems and surgical assistants. CAD/CAM systems have cameras that allow for a highly magnified visualization of the patient's surgical field. Surgical assistants still perform parts of the operation directly. For instance, auxiliary surgical supports assist surgeons with labor-intensive but straightforward tasks, such as holding an endoscope (a medical device with a light attached used to look inside a body cavity or organ) in place.

Conversely, surgical extenders help the surgeon with detailed movements in small anatomical environments. Thus, robot-assisted surgery can allow for more agility and freedom of movement when utilized during laparoscopic surgery (an operation where the physician makes small incisions and inserts tubes/ surgical instruments to manipulate and cut tissue). Currently, laparoscopic surgery is one of the most effective minimally invasive surgical procedures, and physicians can achieve greater control and precision using robot-assisted surgery

Apart from robot-assisted surgery, many robots are utilized in the healthcare industry. Some robots directly assist physicians and nurses, while others maintain the cleanliness and organization of hospitals. There are also companion robots with humanoid features and can even imitate human speech. An interesting type of healthcare robot is an exoskeleton, which are wearable robots that assist patients with physical disabilities. There are treadmill exoskeletons that support the patient's weight while moving the patient's limbs and powered exoskeletons that use motors to assist the patient's movements. Powered exoskeletons allow patients to have increased general control and mobility compared to treadmill exoskeletons, which are typically only used in rehabilitation treatment. Furthermore, there are also tiny robots that can revolutionize current medical practices. These robots can travel into blood vessels to deliver medicine or fight bacteria.

Robotics and Robotics-Assisted Surgery Uses and Applications

The concept of robotics originates from the science fiction works imagined by innovative authors in the early 1900s. In 1958, science fiction became a reality when the first robots were built to assist automobile production. As robotic technology progressed throughout the following decades, robots began to be developed for healthcare usage. The U.S. military was the first to develop robot-assisted surgery and microrobots in the 1970s, initially used for intelligence purposes. In 1985, robot-assisted surgery became highly advanced when the Programmable Universal Manipulation Arm (PUMA) performed a brain biopsy with 0.05 mm accuracy.

Robotics has endless potential within healthcare to address various medical conditions and assist many procedures. For example, exoskeletons are primarily utilized as a rehabilitation treatment for paralyzed patients, such as those who have suffered a spinal cord injury or stroke. Robotic exoskeletons can assist patients in improving their gait and correcting their form. After traditional rehabilitation, 30-40% of stroke survivors still have a limited ability to walk. However, exoskeleton gait training improved patients' walking ability, especially for sub-acute stroke (3-11 weeks after stroke) patients.

Additionally, robots can assist nurses by performing tasks such as creating records, helping patients, performing checkups, and drawing blood. In the future, robots bring the possibility of telenursing, where nurses provide healthcare services remotely through a robot. Disinfection robots are also particularly helpful in hospitals. A practical disinfection method is to use UV-C light, which is 70% more effective than traditional methods. Although UV-C light can effectively prevent bacteria from spreading, it is also harmful to humans. Thus, robots are the perfect tool to prevent the spread of pathogens, especially during pandemics such as COVID-19.

Microrobots that enter a patient's body can navigate to a specific tissue location to deliver drugs, perform microscopic surgery, and take detailed images from within the body. An important application of these microrobots is targeting tumors and preventing the spread of cancerous cells. Due to chemical barriers and blood circulation, other nanomedicines are often hard to reach target cancer cells. However, microrobots are powered by external controls and can actively navigate throughout the bloodstream while protecting the drug from bodily fluids.

Another application of robotics is social robots, which can treat many psychological conditions. For instance, robot companions can reduce symptoms in dementia patients. A study showed that humanoid robot companions could create a calming effect on patients and instigate a strong sense of ownership and attachment. Similarly, social robots can also be used in autism therapy and geriatrics. In addition to providing constant companionship, these robots can automatically record health data for patients continuously.

Robotic surgery is typically utilized in minimally invasive surgical procedures, in which the physician operates using small incisions, but it can also have applications within traditional open surgery. One of the earliest and most widespread applications of robot-assisted surgery is within urology, given the long operative times and the awkward camera position that needs to be held. For instance, robots can perform radical prostatectomy, the removal of the prostate, and other laparoscopic operations. Endoscopic surgery is a minimally invasive surgical procedure where a tube is inserted through an orifice like the mouth or nose. Surgical robots make it possible for physicians to perform highly complex endoscopic surgeries. Physicians can complete cardiac surgery completely using endoscopy with a robot surgery assistant, which was not possible in the past. Robots have also improved mitral valve surgery, which replaces the mitral valve in the heart.

Additionally, robotics also has essential applications within endocrine surgery procedures that remove the thyroid gland (thyroidectomy), parathyroid glands (parathyroidectomy), and adrenal glands (adrenalectomy). The robotic system can provide a 3D magnified view and higher control that can significantly affect the success of a complex procedure. Compared to the current laparoscopic approaches to adrenalectomy, robot-assisted surgery results in shorter operating times and fewer postoperative complications. Next, robots are also utilized in spinal surgeries. Since spinal surgeries require detailed movements within a small area, robot-assisted surgery can be beneficial for performing operations such as placing pedicle screws.

Similarly, robots can assist in arthroplasty procedures by helping to replace joints. In such cases, robot-controlled surgical instruments are highly preferred over the original surgical freehand technique. Thus, robotics clearly has a prominent role in countless types of minimally or invasive surgical operations.

Additionally, robots revolutionized orthopedic surgery in 1992 by assisting medical staff in performing total hip arthroplasty. In 2001, robotics was introduced to pediatric surgery after assisting a surgical operation on a child. Although these technologies were tested and developed in earlier years, many of them were only approved by the FDA in the late 1990s and 2000s. Now surgical robots, including the notorious da Vinci surgical system, are readily available to medical institutions. The da Vinci robot system delivers 3D high-definition views, giving your surgeon a crystal clear view of the surgical area that is magnified 10 times to what the human eye sees. The system is used for prostatectomies, and increasingly for cardiac valve repair, and for renal and gynecologic surgical procedures. In 2020, over 1,000 hospitals installed the da Vinci system, and is projected to increase. The FDA is also continually approving the usage of the da Vinci system in more types of surgery. Given that research on robot-assisted surgery has received plentiful funding, there is no question that advanced developments will occur soon. For instance, future models will incorporate improvements such as haptic feedback, remote telesurgery, and smaller surgical instruments.

Social robot companions and robotic exoskeletons only recently began to be commonly utilized in the 2010s, although the development of these technologies did begin earlier. For instance, robot companions such as Pepper only became available in 2014. Robot companions are currently quite widespread in elderly centers and hospitals, especially in Korea and Japan. New social robots are being launched every year, targeted to specific populations, including patients with disabilities. The elderly population is projected to increase significantly in the decades to come, which will affect caregivers' ability to provide quality care. Thus, it is vital to integrate robotics into current eldercare practices and provide support to caregivers.

Robots can also assist physicians and nurses in repetitive tasks, which increases efficiency. This is already happening in some institutions, including the University of California San Francisco's medical center, which uses robots to transport heavy medical supplies around the facility. However, some areas of robotics, such as exoskeletons, are only utilized by a small number of disabled patients due to their high cost. Currently, purchasing an exoskeleton is the equivalent of investing in a brand-new car with an average price of $45,000. However, it is important to expand the accessibility of exoskeletons in the future to expand its benefits to more of the disabled population.

Robot-assisted surgery is already used by many hospitals worldwide. By 2021, the da Vinci system had performed 10 million surgeries. Additionally, an analysis of 400 randomly selected hospitals in the United States showed that 41% claimed that they used robotic surgery. However, robotic surgery systems are far from cheap, with the da Vinci system costing around 1 million dollars. Even with studies showing that surgical robots reduce overall costs over time, many hospitals cannot afford the initial investment.

Additionally, an important analysis demonstrated that socioeconomic status and race significantly affected a patient's ability to access robotic surgery. Patients were more likely to be in the two highest income brackets, live in metropolitan areas, and have private health insurance. Like the current disparities in healthcare access, the availability of robot-assisted surgery depends on a multitude of societal factors. To make surgical robots available to all patients, addressing the societal barriers that affect their usage is crucial.

The Future of Robotics and Robot-Assisted Surgery

The emergence of robotic technology brings many vital advancements to the healthcare industry. First, exoskeletons can be a powerful tool that can change the lives of disabled patients.

Even with rehabilitation treatments, some patients will remain wheelchair-bound for life. However, exoskeletons can support their bodies and enable patients to stand without assistance. This technology may even eliminate the need for canes and walkers, allowing disabled patients to ultimately reintegrate into their everyday lives when wearing their exoskeletons. Initially, physical therapists would have to physically support patients as they were guided through rehabilitation exercises. With exoskeletons, therapists can teach patients verbally while exoskeletons provide physical support. This would significantly decrease the physical strain on therapists and enable them to provide better treatment to patients.

Similarly, robot companions can provide necessary assistance to overwhelmed caregivers while maintaining the quality of care. These robotic assistants can also contribute to illness prevention and the shift to home care. Since robot companions can stay with patients all around the clock, they can take measurements over an extended period. With this information, doctors would be able to diagnose patients and take preventative measures early on. Instead of staying at a hospital to receive care, patients can stay at home with a robotic assistant, allowing optimal patient comfort.

One of the demographics that would benefit the most from robot companions is the elderly. Because 85% of elderly individuals have a chronic condition, they need access to medical assistance around the clock. However, most elderly patients do not have access to robot companions, especially in the U.S., where only a handful of senior centers have implemented this technology. In Washington DC, a robot companion named SAM lowered costs by 37% and increased patient satisfaction because of its ability to aid 24/7. Robot companions allow patients to feel less only, but they can also help patients take medicine and record health measurements for physicians. Additionally, robotic assistants can be utilized by patients with various conditions. Social robots can care for patients with dementia, autism, and other mental conditions.

During pandemics, robotics can be deployed in the place of front-line workers, allowing doctors to avoid exposure to pathogens. This practical application became especially apparent during the recent COVID-19 pandemic. Throughout the world, robots have been used to monitor patients, take measurements, and run errands in place of physicians. In such times of crises moving forward, robots will be crucial in containing the spread of pandemics and keeping healthcare workers safe. Furthermore, microrobots are also a vital healthcare technology that has countless applications. Not only can they be used to deliver treatment to specific areas of the body, but microrobots can also be used to detect diseases accurately. For instance, capsule endoscopy is a procedure where the patient swallows a microrobot with a small camera, allowing physicians to observe the digestive tract and identify possible infections. By improving diagnosis, healthcare can shift from treatment to prevention.

Robot-assisted surgery provides significant benefits to the healthcare industry compared to other surgical methods. Because of the added control and precision, surgical robots surpass other minimally invasive procedures (such as laparoscopy) in many ways. This precision can provide successful complex surgeries. Surgical robots can also make smaller incisions than surgeons using laparoscopic instruments, providing a cosmetic advantage, decreasing postoperative pain, and speeding up recovery. Additionally, robotics can transform healthcare in rural areas through telemedicine. Physicians and nurses can operate on patients remotely through the robot, potentially opening healthcare access anywhere around the world.

Robotics is utilized in many well-developed healthcare systems around the world. Japan has integrated robotics into many sectors of the country's industry, including healthcare. Since Japan faces a severe elderly wave (a dramatic increase in the elderly population), they have turned to robots to meet the overwhelming demand for elderly care. These robots can recognize emotions, store data, and interact with patients. The new generation of companion bots can remember each patient's personal information better than nurses, allowing for better conversation with patients. Japan is also at the forefront of nursing robotic assistants. Other robots can automatically input medical records and diagnose patients. Additionally, some countries, such as the UK and the U.S., have begun introducing robot companions into healthcare.

Although robotic exoskeletons can already be found in the market, they are hard to access because of their expense. A currently available exoskeleton enables patients in a wheelchair to stand up without other assistance. It sells for $30,000, which is relatively inexpensive compared to other exoskeletons and some medical treatments but can still be prohibitively expensive.

Microrobots were first utilized in medicine at Hong Kong University. Within the U.S., ongoing research on medical microrobots is progressing rapidly. Despite the researchers' progress, microrobots are not used widely in hospitals yet. Despite this, robot-assisted surgery can commonly be found in operating rooms worldwide.

Within the other aspects of the healthcare industry, robotics seems to be slightly underrepresented. For example, despite the useful robots that have been developed to perform the tasks of nurses, there is not a widespread usage of robots in nursing. However, a 2020 study projected that the microrobot market will increase by 78% by 2024. Additionally, the healthcare robotic industry is projected to reach a total worth of $50 billion by 2025, so robotics will likely become more widespread within all healthcare sectors in the years to come.

Robot companions and health assistants should also be increasingly placed within homes. Studies have shown that autonomous robots can effectively care for patients independently within the home. Thus, robots have a vast potential to shift the setting of healthcare from hospitals and medical centers to the comfort of patients' own homes. Additionally, surgical robots open the possibility of widespread healthcare access through telesurgery. Robotic surgery system are being used remotely for surgery and other operations, where the physician operated on a patient from miles away using a robot. Similarly, robotic nurse assistants allow for telenursing. This has enormous humanitarian potential by allowing skilled surgeons and nurses to save the lives of patients in developed countries and rural areas who would not have access to such treatment otherwise.

Risks and Challenges

The use of robotics in healthcare necessitates a discussion of the potential complications and ethical considerations involved. Firstly, there is the possibility of a technology malfunction. For robot-assisted surgery, a survey in 2019 revealed that 26.8% of surgeons had experienced some defect while using the da Vinci surgical system. While this rate may have improved since then, the possibility of a severe malfunction lingers. Thus, scientists need to continue developing new advancements to guarantee the safety of robot-assisted surgery. Other challenges caused by robot-assisted surgery include a high initial cost, more space required, and longer operative times.

Additionally, the haptic feedback (touch) of robot-assisted surgery is not available for in all surgery robots, which may lead to severe mistakes during the operation. Given the relative modernity of surgical robots, there is no standardized training for their use, leading new physicians to be less comfortable when performing robot-assisted surgery. All these complications lead to the importance of informed consent. Patients should be told about the treatment risks, especially given the limited data on robot-assisted surgery.

There is also a possible ethical concern regarding the use of exoskeletons. Although technology isn't quite at this stage yet, robotic exoskeletons have the potential to enhance human abilities beyond normal functionalities. Would it be ethical to allow healthy individuals to utilize exoskeletons to go beyond their physiological limits if this is the case? As exoskeletons become more readily available and begin to advance beyond just rehabilitation, the healthcare industry needs to enforce regulations for its use.

Humanoid robotic companions also raise a plethora of ethical considerations. If robot companions spend more and more time with elderly and disabled patients, the human interaction that patients receive from caregivers will decrease. This may isolate patients and dehumanize their care since they can be treated without human involvement. However, this issue can be quickly addressed by enforcing supervised autonomy (caregivers watch over robots) and maintaining human interaction. Additionally, some robot companions have become almost identical to real humans. This may lead young patients to perceive robots as real humans, distorting their sense of reality. An essential function of robot companions is their ability to take measurements around the clock, giving physicians detailed data to make accurate diagnoses. However, this sort of detailed data collection raises many privacy issues since robots can constantly collect data on every aspect of patients' lives. Thus, physicians must gain informed consent from patients before utilizing robot companions.

Furthermore, as robotic assistants take on more tasks, they have the potential to displace healthcare workers. For instance, fewer nurses may be needed if robots can autonomously take measurements and interact with patients. However, there is generally a shortage of healthcare workers, so robots will likely help relieve overworked physicians and nurses. It is also important for physicians to supervise robots and only allow robots to perform fewer complex tasks, so they are unlikely to displace human workers.

Overall, one of the biggest concerns regarding the development of new technology is the equality of access. Robotic technology is often expensive and only accessible to well-funded hospitals and well-off individuals. This is especially prevalent when looking at the accessibility of robotic exoskeletons in rehabilitative care. Studies have shown that factors including race, socioeconomic status, and location affect a patient's ability to receive robot-assisted surgery. Thus, the healthcare industry needs to implement changes such as a more equitable distribution of care and lower costs to create more accessibility to advanced technology.

Summary

The current and potential applications of robotics in healthcare is exponential. The evidence has made a compelling case that robots can bring significant benefits to physicians, nurses, caregivers, and surgeons, which will increase the overall quality of healthcare. By allowing disabled patients to recover the use of their limbs, robotic exoskeletons can redefine the treatment that disabled patients receive. Similarly, microrobots will revolutionize medical practices by providing a potential alternative to drug treatment and surgery. Additionally, robot companions can address the rising needs of the elderly population and lower healthcare costs in the long term. By staying at the patient's side around the clock, robot companions can take detailed health measurements that allow physicians to make early diagnoses and prevent chronic conditions.

Moreover, robot companions can contribute to the shift to at-home care by allowing patients to receive robotic care from their own homes. Robot companions also have the potential to expand care to a larger population by countering the decreased availability of caregivers and healthcare professionals in some areas of the world. Next, robot assistants can perform menial tasks such as taking measurements, transporting healthcare supplies, and checking in on patients. In this way, robots can fill in the gaps for hospitals with physician shortages while still ensuring the same or even better quality of care. Additionally, these robot assistants can be vital to preventing the spread of disease, an application that has gained traction due to the COVID-19 pandemic.

Robots can be deployed as front-line workers during pandemics, protecting physicians and nurses from risk. Robots can also disinfect hospitals automatically and contain virus outbreaks. Of course, the most important application of robotics in healthcare is robot-assisted surgery. Surgical robots have been shown to improve surgical operations significantly by bringing many benefits, including decreased operative pain, fewer postoperative complications, and greater precision for complicated operations.

Additionally, surgical robots create the possibility of telesurgery, where physicians can perform surgeries remotely from far away. This will revolutionize the availability of surgical treatment by eliminating geographic boundaries. Given the significant impact, robotics can have on the healthcare industry, healthcare stakeholders, leaders, and professionals will begin integrating more robotic technologies into hospitals and patient homes. By doing this, robots will propel the healthcare industry into a progressive future.

Statistics and Trends

- Robot-assisted procedures accounted for 19.1% of all general surgeries in 2021, up from just 1.8% in 2012.
- The use of robotic surgery climbed 12.8% in the first four years after hospitals introduced it.
- In 2021, the global market share for surgical robotics was $7.4 billion, and it's predicted to leap above $29 billion by 2025.

- Among specific procedures tracked, inguinal hernia repair saw the biggest gain in the use of robotic surgery, rising from 0.7% of cases in 2012 to 31.8% in 2021. Other procedures where the use of the robot is up sharply ventral hernia repair, from 0.5% to 22.4%; colectomy, from 2.5% to 16.3%; reflux surgery, from 5.4% to 26.0%; and proctectomy, from 3.1% to 26.7%.
- Robotic surgery statistics demonstrate that over 100,000 robotic-assisted procedures will be performed in 2021 in the U.S.. In that same year, the overall market for robotic surgical systems was valued at over $2.4 billion.
- Statistics show that in 2020, minimally invasive surgeries accounted for approximately 86% of total robotic surgeries performed in the U.S. As more physicians are trained in these techniques. Technology has become more widely available.
- During the past 14 years, more than 1.75 million robotic surgeries have been performed in the U.S. alone across various surgical specialties. Robotic technology replicates the movement of a surgeon's hands, giving us the ability to perform complex, minimally invasive surgeries.
- The global robotic surgery services market is expected to grow from $0.57 billion in 2020 to $0.95 billion in 2021.
- The most widely used clinical robotic surgical system includes a camera arm and mechanical arms with surgical instruments attached to them. The surgeon controls the arms while seated at a computer console near the operating table. The console gives the surgeon a high-definition, magnified, 3-D view of the surgical site.
- Often, robotic surgery makes minimally invasive surgery possible. The benefits of minimally invasive surgery include

fewer complications, such as surgical site infection, less pain and blood loss, quicker recovery, more minor, less noticeable scars, and the act of collecting and analyzing data about a surgeon's every move could put the surgeon under intense, protracted scrutiny.

- The survival rate of patients having minimally invasive surgery compared to patients having open surgery is lower. Over the past two decades, more than 8,061 device malfunctions, 1,391 injuries, and 144 deaths occurred in robotic surgery services.

Chapter 8

3D Printing

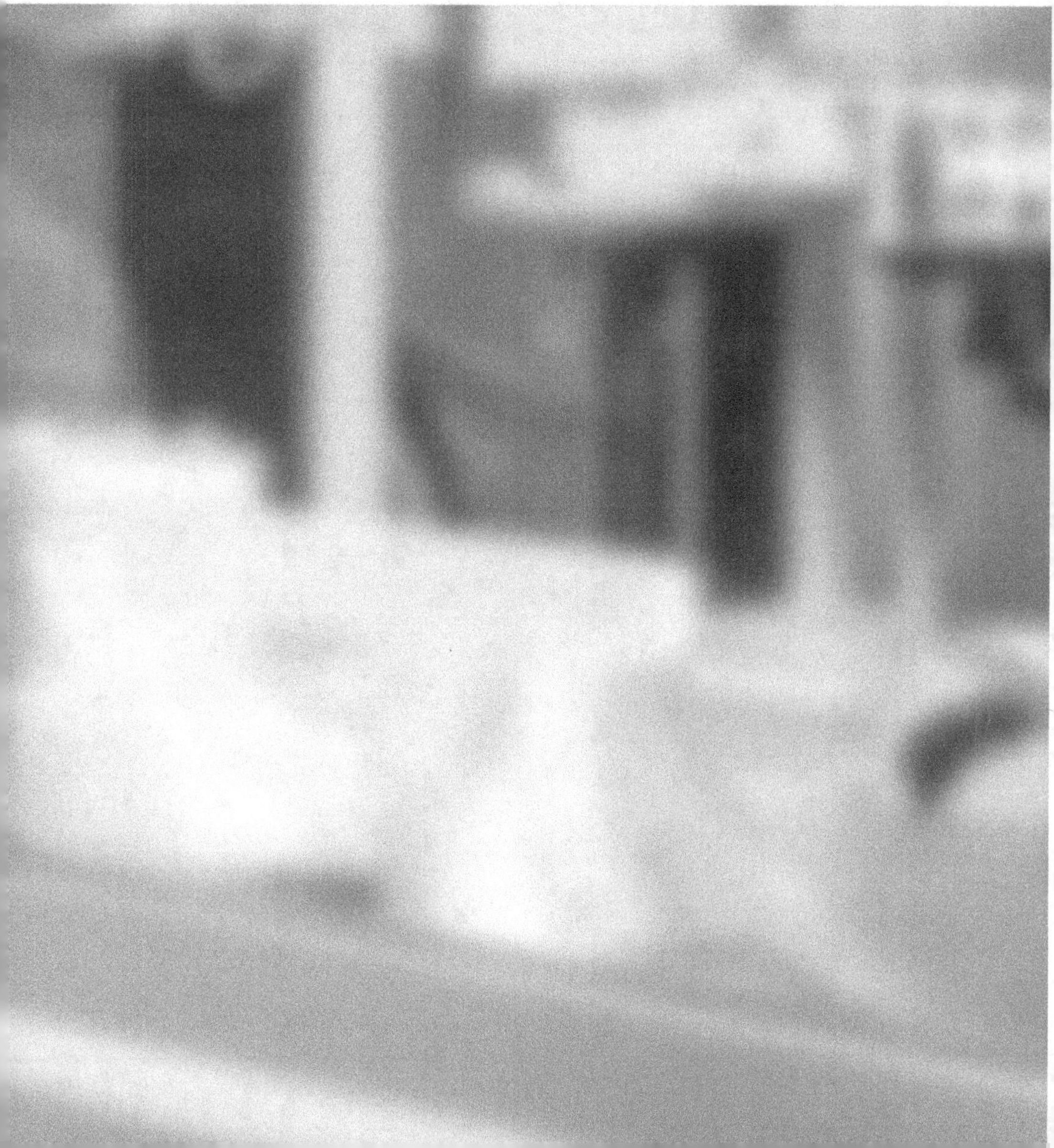

Contents

Introduction

In the last century, 3D printing and bioprinting have undergone substantial transformations. It is a process that could exceedingly revolutionize drug creation and the production of medical equipment in the health and medicine industry. 3D printing and bioprinting are a convergence of biology and engineering technologies, mirroring the clinical need to produce viable biological tissue through printing, regenerative medicine, and materials science advancements. These technological advancements have opened doors to new courses in mimicking the body's processes and new developments in observing the interaction of drugs within the human body. Incremental transformations have been seen in non-invasive data collected from the human body and are a step in the right direction to personalized medication, potentially reducing the number of side effects.

3D and bioprinting are set to be a fundamental part of healthcare. Technology has already infiltrated the surgical field of healthcare, from surgical tools and systems inside the operating rooms to personalized anatomical models. This collaboration is set to reduce healthcare spending and increase personalized care.

What is 3D Printing and Bioprinting?

3D printing has many functions in various industries; however, it has four main applications in the medical field. This technology replaces human organ transplants, speeds up surgical procedures, produces cheaper versions of required surgical tools, and improves the lives of those reliant on prosthetic limbs. Additive manufacturing processes, 3D printing, and bioprinting are accelerating healthcare innovations. For example, 3D printing in healthcare aids in creating tissues and organs, patient-tailored medications, surgical tools, patient-specific surgical models, and custom prosthetics from digital models, or blueprints, of the patient. These models are then created by printing successive layers of the appropriate materials to develop a physical version of the subject.

Bioprinting is an extension of traditional 3D printing. Bioprinting can produce living tissue, bone, blood vessels, and, potentially, whole organs in medical procedures, training, and testing. Similar to 3D printing, bioprinting also uses a digital file as a blueprint to create objects, layer by layer. Contrary to 3D printing, bioprinting utilizes cells and biomaterials to create organ-like structures that allow for cell multiplication. Both processes pose considerable benefits to the healthcare industry.

Uses and Applications of 3D Printing

These developments have assisted cardiac surgeries in improving visualization by creating patient-specific and anatomically detailed conduit bypass models, transcatheter valve and stent, coronary fistulas, as well as teaching and surgical planning models. 3D printing has printed tissues to assist vascular malformations and bone grafts for cleft alveolar osteoplasty and create patient-specific scoliosis braces. This technology has also revolutionized the area of neurosurgery by creating intricate 3D models of individual aneurysms to assist neurosurgeons in performing cerebral aneurysm surgeries and in locating neurotrauma. Furthermore, the translation of MRI data into patient-specific models made possible by 3D printing has improved surgeons' recognition of the brain tumor and its extent amongst the gyral and sulcal patterns and skull features when performing neuro-oncology surgeries.

In orthopedics and orthotics and assistive devices, 3D printing has contributed majorly to creating patient-tailored and customized bio-models, devices, instruments, and implants. This technology has assisted foot, ankle, shoulder, hand, hip, lower limb, scoliosis, and trauma orthopedic surgeries. Additionally, 3D printing technology has vastly aided reconstructions in oral and craniomaxillofacial surgeries. Apart from developing improved teaching and planning models, this additive technology can fabricate mandible models to serve as a template for orbital tumors, visualize bone defects, create orbital floor stamps for orbital floor reconstructions, and customized titanium plates for mandibular reconstructions. Furthermore, the advancement of personalized pharmaceuticals that have been made possible by 3D and bioprinting technologies revolutionizing personalized drug manufacturing. The future of healthcare is patient-tailored, efficient, individualized, and on-demand.

In anatomical and surgical patient-specific models, medical devices and instruments have also benefitted from the technology. 3D printed anatomical models from patient scanned data are becoming increasingly valuable tools in today's personalized, precision medicine practice. New biocompatible medical 3D printing materials have also enabled new surgical tools and techniques to be developed to further improve the clinical experience during surgery. Progressions in manufacturing new medical devices and instruments have also benefited from 3D printing. The ease of use and low cost of in-house 3D printing has also revolutionized product development. Many medical tool manufacturers have adopted the technology to produce brand new medical devices and surgical instruments.

Over 90 percent of the top 50 medical device companies use 3D printing to create accurate prototypes of medical devices and jigs and fixtures to simplify testing. Project engineers of global providers of medical devices are now heavily relying on 3D printing for more transparent communication of designs and a massive reduction in time and costs. This technology has pharmaceutical and medical device development companies gain massive in-house prototype designing and printing capabilities. To date, 3D printing and bioprinting have had immense impacts on creating patient-specific anatomical and surgical models and medical devices and instruments.

3D printing has also benefitted the prostheses, corrective insoles, and orthoses part of healthcare. Simple prostheses are only available in a few sizes. Patients must make do with what fits best, while custom-fit bionic devices designed to mimic the motions and grips of real limbs that rely on muscles in a person's residual limb to control their functions are expensive. In addition, they're only accessible to patients with the best health insurance in developed countries. This particularly affects prostheses for children. Children inevitably outgrow their prostheses and require expensive repairs as children grow and get into adventures. The difficulty is the lack of manufacturing processes that affordably produce custom parts.

The low cost of producing these prostheses and the freedom that comes with custom designs have proved revelatory. Prostheses made with 3D printing can be turned around in as little as one week and then can be reprinted at a much lower cost than their traditional counterparts. Many of the same high financial barriers to treatment seen in prosthetics are also native to fields such as orthoses and insoles. Like many other patient-specific medical devices, custom orthoses are often inaccessible due to their high cost and take weeks or months to manufacture.

Bioprinting offers several applications in tissue engineering and organ printing. The conventional means of treating patients with severe organ failures currently involve using autografts, a graft of tissue from one point to another of the same individual's body, or organ transplants from a donor. Researchers in the fields of bioprinting and tissue engineering are hoping to change that soon and be able to create tissues, blood vessels, and organs on demand. 3D bioprinting refers to additive manufacturing processes to deposit materials known as "bioinks" to create tissue-like structures used in medical fields. Tissue engineering refers to the various evolving technologies, including bioprinting, to grow replacement tissues and organs in the laboratory to treat injury and disease.

There have been exciting breakthroughs in biological materials suitable for 3D printers. Scientists are developing new hydrogel materials that have the same consistency as organ tissue found in the human brain and lungs and can be compatible with various 3D printing processes. Scientists are hoping to be able to implant them onto an organ to act as a scaffold onto which cells would be encouraged to grow.

While bioprinting fully functional internal organs such as hearts, kidneys, and livers still sound futuristic, hybrid 3D printing techniques are rapidly advancing. Soon, building biological matter in laboratory printers is expected to lead to the ability to generate new, fully functional 3D printed organs. Like 3D printing, bioprinting uses a digital file as a blueprint and prints layer by layer. However, this technology creates cells, biomaterials, and organ-like structures that enable cell multiplication. The first step, known as pre-bioprinting, begins with creating a digital file for the printer to utilize as a blueprint. Next, clinicians prepare bioinks, which are live cells mixed with other materials to produce engineered or artificial live tissue.

These bioinks are mainly composed of the cells being used but are often used in tandem with additional materials that wrap the cells, called biopolymer gels. Then in preparation for bioprinting, a live-cell imaging system is utilized to ensure there are enough cells to print a tissue model successfully. Bioprinting begins with developing different tissue types and requires using different types of cells, bioinks, and equipment. Post-bioprinting is the final step, where structures are crosslinked to achieve complete stability. In the future, bioprinting can bring immense impact on a range of application areas and revolutionize organ and drug production.

The Future of 3D Printing

3D printing and bioprinting have made lasting impacts in the healthcare industry. These technologies were mainly used by major manufacturers that could afford expensive materials and printers in the past. Over the last couple of decades, these printing technologies have evolved to become more affordable and available for various industries, such as healthcare. 3D and bioprinting will continue to make immense impacts in the future.

3D printing for orthopedic implants was initially used over a decade ago, with the first 3D-printed implants made around 2007. The technology enables medical practitioners to build improved fitting implants, endure longer, and function better. Today, the technology may be utilized to create a variety of implants, such as spinal, hip, knee, and skull implants. In the future, with design flexibility provided by 3D printing, implants with porous surface structures can be created, allowing for faster integration of a biological bone with the artificial implant.

Using the patient's medical imaging, 3D printing technologies are increasingly employed to create patient-specific models of organs and surgical tools. Surgeons can reduce patients' wait time in the operating room by prepping for surgery with a 3D-printed model. This results in fewer complications and a better long-term outcome for the patient. In the future, 3D printed material and organs will be a mayor part of the medical, research, and educational field.

Personalized surgical equipment is another area where 3D printing is having an effect. 3D printers can be used to create surgical equipment such as forceps, hemostats, scalpel handles, and clamps. Creating bespoke surgical equipment has numerous advantages. In the future, these advancements will allow for faster and less stressful surgeries, improve a surgeon's dexterity, and contribute to better surgical outcomes. Low-cost personalization is a crucial benefit, driving the adoption of 3D printing for medical and dental devices. It has been used for applications of braces, dentures, aligners, restorations, and prosthetics. 3D printing is predicted to make a significant impact in the dental sector. Over the next five years, 3D printing is expected to evolve to the point where it can be used to create clear aligners directly.

3D printing is becoming more popular in hospitals, resulting in personalized healthcare solutions in cardiac surgery to pediatric care. These developments are only the beginning. Many manufacturers will be dedicated to improving healthcare rather than simply selling 3D printers in the future. They will actively participate in medical advisory committees, define regulatory norms, and provide medical-specific services and resources. Some 3D printing technologies have undergone FDA-approved testing. As hospital applications increase, these companies focus on addressing physical requirements while also exploring novel materials and technologies.

3D printing is being used to combat the Covid-19 epidemic. The rapid spread of Covid-19 has put pressure on healthcare systems worldwide, with a surge in demand for crucial medical equipment and supplies. Major firms and people have responded to the Covid-19 issue by assisting in producing critical hospital medical equipment using 3D printers. These technologies will be making immense impacts in the subsequent pandemics to come.

3D printing will create new opportunities in regenerative medicine. There is a severe health problem in terms of organ shortages, as the population lives longer as a result of medical developments. Since 2013, the number of patients in need of an organ transplant has doubled, but the number of available donor organs has barely changed. Regenerative medicine encompasses a wide range of disciplines, including scaffolds, biomaterials, cells, or a mix of biomaterials and cells to manufacture organs for transplantation rather than relying on the present donor model. 3D printing will be able to assist with challenging technological achievements in the sector recently through the production of multilayered things (tissues/organs) using soft biomaterials such as living cells and biomimetic synthetic polymers.

3D printing provides a whole new opportunity to create and prepare individualized medications on both a pharmacy and an industrial scale. When 3D printers are introduced into pharmacies and hospitals, physicians, nurses, and pharmacists will be able to create a dose and delivery system based on the patient's body size, age, lifestyle, and gender.

Bio-printed tissues and organs are already being used to improve clinical trial success rates and will continue to further assist in advancing this field. In the future, researchers can use bioprinting to create fully functional organs made of human cells to assess a drug's efficacy before performing in vivo animal or human experiments. This lowers animal suffering and speeds up the entire research and development process.

Healthcare expenses are always an issue for hospitals and insurance companies alike. 3D printing boosts medical staff efficiency by reducing preoperative planning hours, which helps hospitals cut expenditures on every surgery. Furthermore, hospitals can look to 3D printing plastic replacement components for various devices that frequently require costly replacements. A broken plastic tube or clip might often necessitate the replacement of an entire machine. These parts can be replaced in half a day using 3D printing and $1 resin.

The ability to bioprint organs and tissue patches from a patient's cells reduces the risk of rejection and, in some situations, eliminates the need for organ donors. Researchers will be able to use bioprinting technology in the future to build simple homocellular tissue models for basic research or more complex scaffolds with controlled spatial heterogeneity of physical properties, cellular composition, and extracellular matrix (ECM)/biomolecule structure. The ECM is a complex network composed of several multidomain macromolecules organized in a cell/tissue-specific manner. ECM components join to produce a structurally stable composite that contributes to tissue mechanical properties. Spatially specified gradients of immobilized biomolecules can be created automatically and without contact, reducing the danger of surface cross-contamination and eliminating the need to chemically modify printed proteins or substrates. Bio-printed gradients and biomolecule patterns can help us learn more about how to improve stem cell microenvironments.

This revolutionary 3D printing application has the potential to improve our understanding of complex diseases and produce novel personalized treatments for diseases such as cancer, which currently kills one out of every seven people worldwide. The continued progress and use of this core technology promise to one day allow the creation of bespoke tissue-engineered constructions and "made to order" solid complex organs a reality. The capacity to generate tissue on a chip will enable researchers to explore new regenerative medicine and drug development strategies. Researchers can also study other methods of generating chips by using a 3D bioprinter.

Furthermore, blood vessel bioprinting is a very young medical field. The ability of a bioprinter to create blood arteries is beneficial not just for direct transplantation into patients but also for medication testing and personalized therapy. Researchers have made strides in this sector by printing agarose strands that serve as blood vessels. Instead of dissolving around an existing structure, the researchers discovered that these bio-printed blood arteries could move and form more extensive networks.

Risks and Challenges

Unlocking the full potential of 3D bioprinting for healthcare is not without challenges. Several recent reports have raised concerns regarding the adoption of regenerative medical interventions such as 3D bioprinting into mainstream clinical practice. The bioprinting process requires cells, bio-inks, and bioprinters, each presenting biological, technical, and ethical challenges and uncertainty regarding clinical effectiveness and cost-effectiveness.

While a 3D-printed prosthetic may be classified as Class I, or low risk, the technology has enabled more advanced implants and tools to be produced that encompass Class III, or high risk, medical devices. To certify devices under Class I, manufacturers have to prove that the final product is essentially the same as a device already on the market. For Class II and III medical devices, FDA and other regulatory bodies have yet to issue guidelines on pre-market approval of 3D-printed medical devices. These are innovative products and would likely require modifications to an existing medical regulatory framework.

To date, more than 200 medical devices have been approved by the FDA, most of which fall under Class I medical devices. Patient-specific devices are the most complicated case to regulate. Traditionally manufactured medical devices are standard, one-size-fits-all. Within the healthcare industry, reimbursement describes the payment that a hospital, doctor, diagnostic facility, or other healthcare providers receive for providing a medical service.

As such, the translation of 3D bioprinting into mainstream clinical practice will be presented with significant challenges. Speculated roles of 3D bioprinting in surgery include the production of de novo root organogenesis for transplantation and the use of autologous cellular material for personalized medicine. The research that stems from bioprinting is fascinating. While there has been considerable advancement in knowledge and gains made from the ability to bio-print bones, skin, blood vessels, cartilage, and even organs, there's still much more progress before many of these practices are adapted into medicine. In the case of bioprinting and skin, researchers hope to have the science ready within five years for soldiers who experience extensive burns in combat.

Furthermore, few human studies have shown effective clinical translation of tissue-engineered structures. There is still some uncertainty about how autologous cells would behave. Because implants contain biological components, integration and interactions with hosts are more unpredictable than with currently employed stents, pacemakers, and artificial joints. Genotype differences in patients will influence processes such as cell migration, post-printing phenotype, carcinogenic potential (especially in immortalized cell populations), and dysregulated differentiation, such as fat-derived stem cells creating ectopic bone.

Clinical trial designs are also proven to be a challenge. Indeed, the few trials using tissue-engineered constructions have been in patients with a terminal disease, when such "last resort" choices are frequently regarded as "more ethical," despite the risk of problems. In the case of skeletonized trachea from cadavers can be seeded with patient mesenchymal stem cells and used in surgery.

It is difficult to portray the patients' clinical urgency and obtain necessary ethical permission. This trial was described as a last resort alternative and a final opportunity at a lifesaving intervention, which aided in obtaining ethical approval to administer the treatment to patients. Another difficulty in organizing clinical trials is that patients cannot withdraw after implantation, and permission for trial inclusion is difficult when the number of problems is unknown.

Summary

In the medical field, 3D Printing has four main applications. This technology replaces human organ transplants, speeds up surgical procedures, produces cheaper versions of required surgical tools, and improves the lives of those reliant on prosthetic limbs. Bioprinting technology's broad applications have already been demonstrated globally, resulting in the creation of unique constructs ranging from arteries and composite tissue to organoids and sophisticated cellular and tissue models for pharmacological, cosmetic, and experimental testing. Personalized, precision medicine is on the rise. New tools and advanced technologies bring doctors closer to patients, delivering treatments and devices customized to serve each unique individual better. Advances in medical 3D printing technology have made tremendous contributions to fields throughout healthcare. For patients, new tools and therapeutic methods developed through 3D printing can bring new degrees of comfort and personalization to treatment. For doctors, this newly accessible technology allows for a greater understanding of complex cases and provides new tools that can ultimately result in a higher standard of care.

From surgical planning models to 3D printed vasculature and bioreactors, 3D printing in healthcare is taking off, and many medical professionals are excited about the potential of this technology in medicine. The introduction of human cells and biocompatible materials into the 3D printing techniques are expected to result in a paradigm change for surgery, allowing for the 3D printing of living tissue and organs. To fully realize the potential of 3D printing in surgery, doctors must stay current on breakthroughs in the field, identify niches where this technology might be employed, and promote its incorporation into mainstream surgical practice. With incremental advances in 3D printing and bioprinting expected over the next century, the impact on the future of surgery could be transformational.

Statistics and Trends

- 3D Printing in healthcare was valued at $1.12 Billion in 2019 and is projected to reach $3.93 Billion by 2027, growing at a rate of 17.1%.
- The global 3D printing material market is forecast to expand at 26% over the duration of 2021 to 2031. According to the study, 3D printing materials is gaining traction in healthcare owing to its utility in creating artificial organs and cells.
- The medical applications for 3D printing consist of prosthetics, implants, orthopedic and orthotic devices (e.g., joint replacement, splints), and surgical instruments custom-made for a patient's specific anatomy.
- 3D printing has also been used for designing anatomical mechanisms that are required for respiratory, spinal, craniofacial, and dental repair. By implementing 3D

printing, it offers benefits to the patients where the patient is at comfort and will be under anesthesia for less time.

- Today, technology can make a broad range of implants such as spinal, hip, knee, and skull implants. It's estimated that 6,00,000 implants had been produced with 3D printing in 2019 and by 2027, is expected to increase to 4 million.
- 3D printing is used for the development of new surgical cutting and drill guides, prosthetics as well as the creation of patient-specific replicas of bones, organs, and blood vessels.
- 3D printing of models affords further insights into pathological changes, as well as a visualization of patient-specific organ anatomy.
- 3D bioprinting offers the potential to create functional, living, 3D human tissues of particular organs. These 3D tissues provide much more accurate mimicry to reality, resulting in much more predictive results for drug candidates
- Since 2013, the number of patients requiring an organ has doubled, while the actual number of available donor organs has barely changed. Although many problems need to be solved for complex organs (such as the heart or liver) to be 3D bioprinted and transplanted into a patient, simple organs such as the bladder have been transplanted.
- 3D printing is already being implemented to produce pharmaceuticals by many U.S. companies.
- Prosthetics have historically been expensive. Certain organizations have been designing prosthetics that can be 3D printed from commercially available, affordable desktop printers.

Chapter 9

Healthcare Trackers, Wearables and Sensors

Contents

Introduction

The invention of the first pedometer (step-counter) is credited to horologist and inventor Abraham-Louis Perrelet. However, it has been suggested that Thomas Jefferson also later produced his own mechanical pedometer, improving on Perrelet's original design. As we know them today, fitness trackers first surfaced in 1965 with the Manpo-kei, which translates to "10,000 steps meter" and was invented by Dr. Yoshiro Hatano, a Japanese professor at the Kyushu University of Health and Welfare. Dr. Hatano was then researching how to combat obesity. He hypothesized that 10,000 steps per day would provide the proper caloric intake and calorie expenditure balance to maintain a healthy body. Today, fitness trackers still use this 10,000-step benchmark. Since the 1960s, fitness tracking devices and their technology have developed rapidly, from the introduction of wireless heart rate monitors in watches in the 1980s to mobile phones that incorporate 3D accelerometers that measure movement and vibration in a three-dimensional space.

Healthcare trackers and sensors are becoming widespread in various applications, from healthcare to biomedical monitoring systems. They enable continuous measurement of critical biomarkers for medical diagnostics, physiological health monitoring, and evaluation. With the increase of the global elderly population, various diseases are becoming more prevelent. The need for point-of-care (POC) diagnosis and real-time monitoring of long-term health conditions are also growing. Accessories, integrated clothing, body attachments, and body inserts are some results of the evolution of wearable devices. The electronics, biocompatible materials, and nanomaterials developed over the past decades have led to implantable devices, which can be used for diagnosis and prognosis through small sensors and biomedical devices and significantly improve the quality and efficacy of medical services. Their development will only continue within the next decade, causing changes in care sites and the arrangement of delivery systems.

In many cases, the quality of care will be improved, and patients can be managed in their homes. Hospitals will operate differently, more safely, and more efficiently. As these advances are costly, they will remain irrelevant in many parts of the world, which would benefit the most from increased vaccine development instead of new sensors. There is a significant contrast between the upper socioeconomic classes with access to sophisticated medical technologies and the lower socioeconomic classes that continue to bear unnecessary morbidity and mortality. This shows the importance of placing health inequity as a top priority.

What are Healthcare Trackers, Wearables, and Sensors?

The advancement of wearable technology and growing demand from consumers to take control of their health has influenced the medical industry, including insurers, providers, and technology companies, to develop more wearable devices such as smartwatches and wearable monitors. Healthcare trackers and sensors are quite similar in nature. Healthcare trackers are devices that collect and analyze various data points related to one's health. They can track a wide variety of health-related data, such as the number of steps one has taken throughout the day, calorie intake, heart rate, blood pressure, sleep patterns, and more. Wearable

ECG (Electrocardiogram) monitors are on the cutting edge of consumer electronics, and what sets these monitors apart from some smartwatches is their ability to measure electrocardiograms or ECGs.

For example, some ECG monitors can measure an electrocardiogram, send the reading to the user's doctor, and detect atrial fibrillation. It's also able to track pace, distance, elevation, and automatic tracking for walking, running, swimming, and biking. Similarly, healthcare sensors are implanted or digestible devices which measure health parameters and vital signs according to the patient's needs. Because of the nature of these devices, they can make telemedicine and preventative care easier as they bring healthcare into the patient's home.

Biosensors are up-and-coming wearable medical devices radically different from wrist trackers and smartwatches. A wearable biosensor is a self-adhesive patch that allows patients to move around while collecting data on their movement, heart rate, respiratory rate, and temperature. Research shows that this wearable device registered an 89% reduction in patient deterioration into preventable cardiac or respiratory arrest. This demonstrates the ability wearables have to improve patient outcomes and possibly reduce staff workload.

Smart sensors are increasingly offering novel solutions to several relevant challenges in healthcare, like early detection of pathologies and minimally invasive management and prevention of high-burden diseases like cardiovascular diseases and cancer. The development of miniaturized and lightweight, intelligent sensor-based systems may be vital in enabling more rapid growth of unobtrusive and unsupervised approaches to home rehabilitation and the continuous monitoring of a patient's status.

Healthcare Tracker and Sensor Uses and Applications

Healthcare trackers and sensors are currently being used to help prevent diseases and maintain health by monitoring physical activity and calorie intake. These healthcare devices can also directly impact clinical decision-making and be used for disease management. Wearable technologies enable the continuous monitoring of human physical activities and behaviors and physiological and biochemical parameters during daily life.

The various healthcare sensor grades currently being used range from consumer to clinical to research-grade devices. Data from these sensors have been used in a wide range of tasks, including tracking gait (a person’s way of walking), detecting atrial fibrillation (irregular and often very rapid heart rhythm), and monitoring blood glucose. Wearable mechanical sensors usually utilize inertial measurement units (IMUs) to estimate a subject's translational and rotational motion, applied forces, and surrounding magnetic field. IMUs function by using biaxial or triaxial accelerometers to measure movement. They use gyroscopes to measure rotation and relative position and magnetometers. Accelerometers are most common in wearables, but gyroscopes are appropriate when it is necessary to differentiate acceleration due to gravity versus acceleration due to movement. Other technologies used are global positioning systems, which can detect exact positioning during movement, and altimeters, which can continually correct for drift errors. Wearable pressure sensors have also become increasingly common to track forces exerted on or by the body.

With healthcare devices currently leading to many benefits in the medical field and healthcare industry, it is crucial to think about what the future holds for these technologies and healthcare in general. It is predicted that healthcare trackers and sensors will provide more accurate measurements of physical status and physiological parameters in more convenient ways. Soon, they will influence different aspects of health care, such as prevention through activity tracking and stress monitoring, diagnosis through early detection technology, and disease management. Newer technologies are continuously being developed and eventually released into the wearables market. One example of a developed device is a wearable bandage and microneedle electrochemical sensing platform that can detect the presence of the tyrosinase enzyme biomarker on the skin to rapidly screen for melanoma. Other technologies still under development include skin patches, smart contact lenses, implantable and ingestible devices, head-mounted devices, and E-textiles. As the technology strays further away from wrist-mounted healthcare devices, it is approaching a new era of technology that is still considered futuristic. Healthcare technologies' ever-evolving and exciting possibilities are endless, from smart pills to bio-sensitive ink.

Healthcare trackers and sensors are currently being used when an individual wants to prevent any future illnesses or track and maintain their health. They can be used during pregnancies and menstrual cycles and for individuals with diabetes who need to monitor their diet strictly. In a study the Chronicle Diabetes system was reviewed by diabetes educators. The Chronicle Diabetes system transfers tracker-collected self-monitoring information from patients to diabetes educators. Five themes emerged from this study. First, researchers were enthusiastic about the ability to view diet and physical activity data in the system, but they did have concerns. Second, researchers valued viewing detailed dietary macronutrients and activity data, but they preferred different details depending on the patient's specific needs, conditions, and behavioral goals. Third, and most importantly, all researchers liked the integration of mobile phone-collected data into the Chronicle Diabetes system, preferably with current EHR systems. They also realized that a health care team and a central EHR system were needed to share data with other providers. Lastly, the researchers also wanted more advanced features for the app and connected interface.

Wearable biosensors are essential for the widespread field of health informatics because they can track continuous data. Healthcare trackers and sensors are also used in hospital environments to monitor patients remotely. These healthcare technologies can also be used when an individual's health must be monitored in real-time to prevent various chronic and acute diseases or to bring awareness to their lifestyle. Analyzing this data can show patterns of data points, outliers, and the onset of poor health, allowing for intervention. Typically, patients only have their blood pressure, and temperature measured once every year or two during a visit to the doctor. This information is ignored unless the results are outside of the normal range. Healthcare trackers can lead to a future where this health data is continuously monitored. In the future, healthcare trackers and sensors will serve a different purpose. Instead of simply trying to prevent illness, these healthcare devices will additionally provide intervention and treatment for existing illnesses.

Today, healthcare trackers and sensors are being used in clinics and hospitals, gyms, and work environments to monitor heart rate and activity, and weight loss programs and initiatives, as patients like to see quantifiable results of their progress. Diabetic patients also use them to track insulin levels throughout the day. Web-based electronic health records platform will let physicians access data from fitness trackers, glucose monitors, and heart monitors uploaded by the patients themselves. This is an attempt to create a one-stop-shop for health information, rather than having to manually report data from the trackers to a hospital or physician.

Future patient monitoring and clinical care will be based on efficient and affordable solutions for healthcare trackers and sensors, enabling remote and long-term patient monitoring in homes and communities previously inaccessible. In the future, results collected by this healthcare technology at home can quickly be sent to the individual's physician at a hospital to diagnose, prevent, or treat an illness. The gap between home care and clinical care will finally close with the strides taken to advance healthcare trackers and sensors. Because of these technologies, health care will become more accessible to patients who live in remote areas or are homebound. Patients will not need to travel to meet with experts and can transmit their data or have virtual visits with nurse practitioners. Other types of caregivers can also benefit from using the data from healthcare trackers and sensors to track the care of elderly parents and other homebound patients.

The Future of Healthcare Trackers and Sensors

A variety of individuals and facilities are currently using healthcare trackers and sensors, including patients in hospitals and clinical environments, participants in study projects and research initiatives, athletes and personal fitness enthusiasts, patients with diabetes, cardiac, or respiratory problems, and rehabilitation facilities. Individuals who want to track their health or gain insight into their lifestyle through measurements of health factors also use these devices. Despite the increased use of activity trackers, little is known about how they can be used in healthcare settings. A study with chronic Illness aimed to support healthcare professionals and patients by embedding an activity tracker in the daily clinical practice of a specialized mental healthcare center and gaining knowledge about the implementation process. An action research design lets healthcare professionals and patients learn how and when they can use an activity tracker. Therapists identified opportunities to embed activity trackers into their clinical reasoning and engage patients in their treatment. Based on their expertise and experiences, therapists had clear ideas about who could benefit from activity trackers. They were able to formulate specific exclusion criteria accordingly. With multiple iterations, the action research approach was needed to support professionals and embed activity trackers into their daily clinical practice within a specialized mental healthcare center.

Since healthcare trackers and sensors will mainly be geared towards treatment in the future, those with underlying illnesses will find them more valuable down the road. A recent review of 31 different studies shows that more than 60% of older adults were interested in the future use of a wearable devices for improving physical and mental health. Still, not many were currently using wearable devices because of a general lack of awareness among the older generations. The study indicated that older populations could benefit from using tracking devices, but more work should be done to increase awareness of this technology. Healthcare trackers and sensors are expected to contribute significantly to the elderly population's healthcare and medical costs and the development of personalized medical care. Though patients are more digitally savvy today, and many expect their nurse practitioners to use data they have personally tracked when receiving care, the line between consumer healthcare trackers, sensors, and medical devices is beginning to blur.

Healthcare trackers and sensors continuously monitor physical activities, behaviors, and physiological and biochemical parameters. They are currently being used to help prevent diseases and maintain health by monitoring physical activity and calorie intake. These healthcare devices can directly impact clinical decision-making and be used for patient and disease management. As individuals can see their health-related data collected over a specific period with healthcare trackers and sensors, they can effectively build healthier habits to prevent diseases. Additionally, consumers embracing healthcare trackers, sensors, and wearable technologies to track personalized data have recently started the Quantified Self (QS) movement. QS refers to individuals using self-tracking tools to help them understand their bodies and minds to examine and act on this information. Single devices such as smartwatches that can monitor an extensive range of personal medical data, including heart rate, physical activity, and sleep patterns, have helped expand this movement and use of personalized data.

In the future, these technologies will serve the purpose of not only preventing but also treating existing diseases as well. For example, smart contact lenses can monitor physiological information about the eyes and tears non-invasively to monitor glucose levels. Diabetes patients can use this technology to track the amount of glucose present in their bloodstream. If the glucose levels get too high or low, the patient and their physician will be notified, so the patients can get the immediate care they need without using a lancing device to prick their finger. Additionally, future healthcare trackers and sensors have the potential to benefit those in need of increased physical activity, such as older adults and those who face significant health challenges. In a qualitative study patients with a chronic disease were positive regarding activity trackers in general. Patients with chronic illnesses perceive activity trackers as motivating them to be more physically active and reach daily activity goals. Patients and those registered for clinical trials can benefit from these technologies simply because of their preventive and predictive nature.

Healthcare trackers and sensors are improving health by preventing and diagnosing diseases, allowing individuals to maintain their health, and forming healthy habits. The accuracy and precision of the selected fitness trackers are reasonable and can indicate the average level of activity and thus the average energy expenditure. In addition, a qualitative study conducted on breast cancer survivors' experiences with an activity tracker integrated into an exercise program revealed that wearing the tracker raised their lifestyle awareness. The fitness trackers motivated them to be physically active and creating more awareness of their sedentary lifestyles. As a result, breast cancer patients could consciously change their daily habits to become healthier.

The advances in the development of wearable and remote monitoring devices are growing exponentially. These devices will soon change the practice of medicine and the performance of clinical research. These platforms will conveniently provide more accurate measurements of physical status and physiologic parameters and quickly influence different healthcare aspects. For example, primary care clinicians and cardiologists have already begun seeing patients with self-detected arrhythmia.

Researchers report the value of healthcare trackers and sensors when used as a secondary diagnostic tool for preventable and chronic diseases such as depression, Parkinson's disease, and sleep apnea. These devices can also provide instant feedback for patients with obesity, anxiety, panic disorders, posttraumatic stress disorders, and asthma, which may help improve outcomes. With faster feedback and an individualistic approach, patients may be more likely to use healthcare trackers and sensors to track data than static or paper methods.

Risks and Challenges

Many challenges are associated with implementing healthcare trackers and sensors into the healthcare industry and medical practices. Most advanced healthcare trackers and sensors are still in their prototype stages and have issues like security, ethics, and user acceptance, which need to be addressed. Additionally, there have not been enough studies to prove the accuracy and precision of these trackers. Many medical professionals have also been slow to embrace the concept of patient-generated data, partly because many are skeptical of the information they don't collect themselves and because many consumer-grade apps and devices aren't approved by the U.S. Food and Drug Administration. Security and patient privacy are other issues concerning doctors and other patient advocates. An internet-based system might not be secure and, intentionally or not, could lead to a breach of patient privacy. Some additional challenges picked up by participants in a study utilizing healthcare trackers and sensors that were most dominant include ease of use, physical design and aesthetics, data management, integration and sharing, and data accuracy.

Another critical problem with healthcare trackers and sensors is user privacy. With the innovations and growth of healthcare trackers and sensors, this may be reversed in the future, and people will have more sensors in and on their bodies.

Summary

Healthcare trackers have come a long way since Abraham-Louis Perrelet and Thomas Jefferson's rudimentary pedometers. Individuals are currently using them to prevent illnesses and maintain health. Many individuals use these devices, but hospitals and other facilities also use them. Healthcare trackers and sensors allow for continuous monitoring of activities and behaviors previously only checked infrequently. Because of the constant and massive amount of data generated by them, healthcare trackers and sensors are currently improving their users' health and general wellness. However, as with a lot of new technology, especially technology connected to the internet, security poses a potential risk. Most trackers and sensors are still prototypes and have yet to be entirely accepted by users. Nevertheless, their future is very bright. Continuous, non-invasive tracking creates much more current, accurate, and plentiful data than traditional methods, and these benefits of healthcare trackers and sensors will continue to improve in their function as disease prevention and intervention, especially for communities with less access to traditional healthcare.

The wearable healthcare technology market is surging, and its maturation will put more wearable technology in the hands of consumers and healthcare facilities. The number of health and fitness app users will stay above 84 million through 2022. This upward trend in wearable fitness technology will influence the decision of insurers, health providers, and companies to take advantage of the benefits of wearable health monitoring devices. Insurers can lessen the rising cost per patient by using wearables to increase customer lifetime value. Wearable technology incentivizes behavior that reduces hospital visits and readmissions due to poorly managed personal health (75% of users agree that wearables help them engage with their health.) U.S. consumer use of wearables increased from 9% to 33% in just four years, and this number will continue to grow as wearable technology becomes more conventional and affordable. Moreover, device connectivity will expand as more accurate wearable sensors are developed, opening the door for insurers and employers to influence healthy lifestyles and boost profitability.

Statistics and Trends

- Nearly half (45%) of Americans have at least tried digital health products such as fitness trackers or mobile health apps.
- Health app users are more likely to be younger, with adults under the age of 55 about twice as likely (24-25%) as those 55 and older (12%) to use them.
- The wearable healthcare technology market is surging, and its maturation will put more wearable technology in the hands of consumers and U.S. businesses. The number of health and fitness app users will stay above 84 million through 2022.
- Wearable technology incentivizes behavior that reduces hospital visits and readmissions due to poorly managed personal health – 75% of users agree that wearables help them engage with their own health.
- Companies are also seeing benefits in offering wearable healthcare technology to employees. Healthier corporate culture is shown to reduce employee turnover. Eemployers who offer five or more well-being 'best practices' had an average turnover of 18%, compared to 29% for those that offer two or fewer.
- U.S. consumer use of wearables increased from 9% to 33% in just four years, and this number will continue to grow as wearable technology becomes more conventional.
- Device connectivity will expand as more accurate wearable sensors are developed, opening the door for insurers and employers to influence healthy lifestyles and boost profitability.

Chapter 10

Medical Tricorder

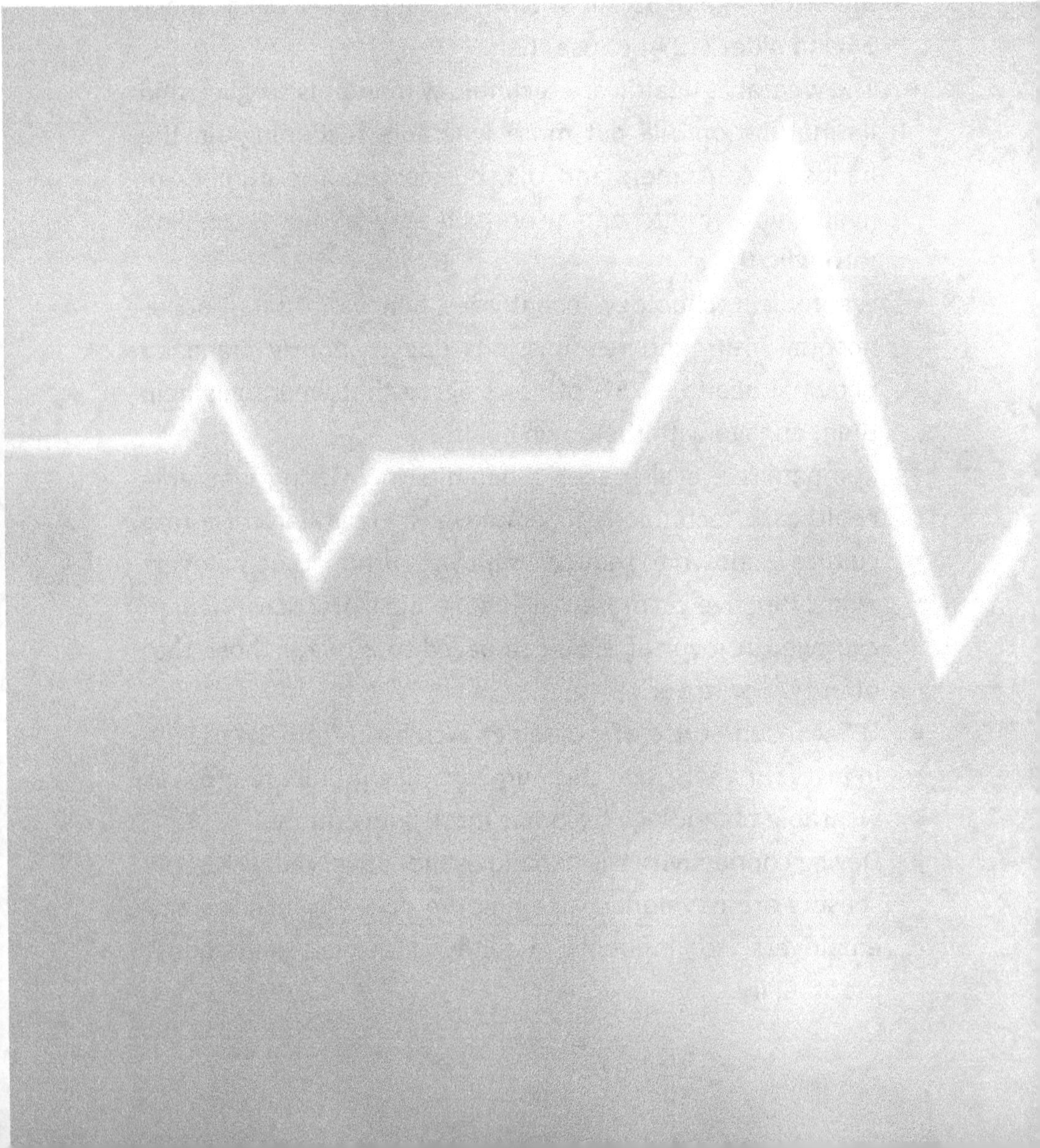

Contents

Introduction

Every healthcare professional's dream is to have one device to diagnose and analyze every disease. A medical tricorder is a portable handheld device used to scan a patient and immediately show vital signs, health indicators, disease, and even make a diagnosis. The original medical tricorder appeared on Star Trek in 1966 as a science fiction scanner. It was a calculator-sized device used to scan a patient. It sensed, recorded, and computed biological data to generate an instant diagnosis, hence the name tricorder. This sci-fi device is the inspiration for today's tricorder. The advantages of a medical tricorder are numerous. Like a Swiss army knife, it is a portable handheld device, and it has multiple functions, such as taking basic vital measurements and diagnosing medical conditions within seconds.

With the exponential progress in healthcare technology, devices that were once a fantasy of sci-fi enthusiasts now exist. For example, currently available is a palm-sized device that can measure heart rate, oxygen saturation, temperature, blood pressure, EKG (electrocardiogram, which records the electrical signal from your heart), and other metrics. Other companies are also working on similar devices with cameras for telemedicine to measure multiple vital parameters. Another device already on the market can measure a wide range of parameters like respiratory rate, heart rate, skin temperature, body position, activity levels, sleep cycles, gait (a person's pattern of walking), stress levels, and more.

Modern tricorders do not yet resemble those seen on Star Trek however. The designs feature several sensors and modules that collect biological data and connect to mobile apps powered by machine learning and artificial intelligence (AI). They are used to diagnose specific conditions, which they do in a relatively non-invasive manner. In the future, they can be expected to be used to diagnose all types of conditions less invasively and with greater convenience.

What are Medical Tricorders?

In 2012, XPRIZE, a non-profit foundation that hosts public competitions to fuel technological developments that will benefit humanity, launched the Qualcomm Tricorder XPRIZE competition. It promised the biggest medical prize in history of $10 million to be divided between three teams that would create a mobile device weighing five pounds or less that could diagnose thirteen diverse diseases better than or equal to a group of specialized physicians. The goal of the medical tricorder was to diagnose whooping cough, hypertension, mononucleosis, shingles, melanoma, HIV, and osteoporosis. In addition, it should be able to continuously monitor the five main vital signs: heart rate, respiratory rate, blood pressure, oxygen saturation, and body temperature. None of the 312 teams that participated in the competition successfully produced such a device. However, XPRIZE awarded prizes to the top three performers, two finalists, and four semi-finalists to further develop and commercialize their prototypes. The usefulness and desire for a medical tricorder have become even more evident over the last decade as their funding is in billions of dollars. The ambition to break through into this multi-billion-dollar market has spurred a race to bring to market the science-fiction device that promises to be within reach in our lifetime.

Today, physicians use many different instruments to determine a patient's health. Some are small and can be used by consumers, like thermometers, while others require a healthcare practitioner's expertise, like a stethoscope or EKG. Each medical tool can currently evaluate one specific area of health without interpreting the results. Medical tricorder researchers, engineers, and scientists are designing devices that collect information and analyze all relevant data for a reliable diagnosis of many conditions. For now, tricorder sensors are smaller, less invasive, and more comprehensive than other diagnostic techniques. Also, diagnostic algorithms are more accurate for some diseases and are smaller and more portable than standard devices. The smaller these components are, the more convenient for the user. The smarter and more reliable they are, the more autonomous and efficient healthcare will become.

Medical Tricorder Uses and Applications

The prospects for producing a medical tricorder have been boosted enormously due to the spread of smartphones. More than six billion smartphones are in usage worldwide, capable of performing as powerful, internet-capable pocket computers. Even with no additional hardware or software, a phone can be a valuable medical device. A smartphone can become an even more powerful tool for monitoring a patient's overall health by connecting hardware sensors. For home use, some tricorders consist of sensors that connect to a smartphone via a mobile application, which collects vital signs, presents surveys and questionnaires, and includes video conferencing and text messaging. The physician has access to a medical dashboard to remotely record thousands of patients' healthcare information. Cloud-based algorithms analyze the signals and determine the likelihood that the patient's condition needs more attention. Some systems, aided by AI, can notify a physician if a patient experiences changes in a particular condition or needs immediate assistance. For example, this remote digital platform enables physicians to monitor patients with chronic illnesses and postoperative cardiac patients.

This is just one notable example. The use and interest in remote patient monitoring and more comprehensive telemedicine are increasing, especially in the age of the COVID-19 pandemic. Another company introduced a remote patient monitoring platform that features a pinnacle in sensor technology: one handheld device that measures heart rate, respiration rate, blood oxygen level, and temperature. It also listens to the heart, lungs, and abdomen and looks inside the nose, throat, mouth, and ears. Furthermore, it inspects skin and can perform an EKG, making the home use tricorder a smaller, more autonomous device.

Medical tricorders can also turn smartphones into digital first-aid kits. One example of this is an otoscope (a device for looking inside the ear) that clips onto a smartphone. Physicians can use it for diagnosis and visual record-keeping, or parents can use it to transmit images to pediatricians for the remote diagnosis of children's ear infections, which cause millions of visits to the doctor each year. Other examples include testing for the presence of strep throat, flu, or other types of upper-respiratory infections. While these results are encouraging, one must understand that medical algorithms for treatment and diagnostic testing (MATD) were designed to diagnose a specific problem and not pick a diagnosis out of every possible condition. The algorithm behind WebMD or Google performs far worse than doctors at correctly diagnosing a disease when given the same information.

Today, Star Trek's tricorder remains science fiction. Every component necessary to make a tricorder a handheld, comprehensive medical, or consumer diagnostic device has yet to be developed to that level. They are rapidly advancing, but they all have a long way to go, some only in their technological infancy. Even those innovations in adolescence have limited implementation in the lives of physicians, patients, and consumers. However, these realities do not make the advent of the tricorder any less likely. Currently, full medical tricorders remain in development. Those produced in the past shared a general design of separate sensors and modules that non-invasively record biological data, which they transmit to a mobile app powered by algorithms, machine learning, and AI that can diagnose certain diseases.

One of the newest medical tricorders is not portable and consists of four separate modules. It can measure blood pressure and has a chest sensor that continuously monitors EKG, heart rate and rhythm, body temperature, a spirometer that performs pulmonary function tests, and a particularly innovative wrist sensor for continuous monitoring of pulse, oxygen, and heart rate, and blood pressure. This device also uses a non-invasive sensor that monitors glucose, hemoglobin, and white blood counts. This device uses machine learning algorithms to reliably diagnose a total of 34 diseases using the data collected. It is not currently available on the market as it is still in the research and design stages and needs to prove the requirements set by the Federal Drug Administration (FDA) and other U.S. agencies.

Another smartphone-connected tricorder underway uses high–powered microscopes with smartphones to analyze swab samples and photos of skin lesions. These sensors could pick up abnormalities in DNA or detect antibodies and specific proteins. Many technologies could be attached to a smartphone to augment it, like an ultrasonic probe. Such developments will have profound implications. Much like mobile phones did in the past, these devices will help physicians reduce their workload and, more importantly, help them provide better, more personalized care. The goal is to create a mobile platform that will enable people to diagnose conditions, including diseases as varied as pneumonia, diabetes, and sleep apnea, without relying on physicians or nurses.

Another company's medical tricorder uses a Bluetooth-enabled scope set to perform blood, urine, and breath tests and monitor vital signs. While physicians are using medical tricorders, others are geared toward consumers. The consumer medical tricorder-based sensor technology and diagnostic algorithms are used for comprehensive remote patient monitoring by physicians and researchers. Many companies research, develop, and sell separate healthcare trackers and sensors. Still, most are innovative in that they bring sensors to consumers instead of doing everything with one single device. For example, some healthcare providers already send out text messages to patients' mobile phones, enabling them to take their medication, renew their prescriptions, order medications, and schedule and remind patients of appointments.

The Future of Medical Tricorders

Current consumer wearable trackers monitor heart rate, count steps, calories, stress levels, and even sleep. Innovations in sensor technology in healthcare are miniaturized and put into consumer electronics. As new devices come to market, consumers will have access to powerful, multi-functional wearables.

In 2017, Cloud DX started selling its Connected Health platform. It consists of FDA-cleared medical devices, including Pulsewave for blood pressure, a wireless weight scale, a pulse oximeter, a thermometer, and a glucose meter. All these devices use Bluetooth to connect to a mobile application on a tablet. The mobile application collects vital signs, presents surveys and questionnaires, delivers content like articles and video clips, and includes two-way video conferencing and text messaging features. A web-based clinical dashboard allows doctors, nurses and AI to monitor up to thousands of patients remotely, seeing their vital signs and symptoms in near real-time. AI analyzes this data to determine negative changes. If those changes occur, a message is sent to the patient's care team that notifies them that the patient might need assistance. According to an SEC filing report, measurements had been taken from tens of thousands of patients.

The COVID-19 pandemic demonstrated the utility of at-home diagnostic technology. Consumers will benefit from fewer in-person visits to a doctor or hospital depending on the severity and length of the pandemic and the new social distancing culture. Sensors will get smaller while collecting more physiological data, less invasively. Currently, there is a consumer market for wearable sensors. Tricorder technologies promise to solve healthcare's biggest challenges. Sensors increasingly allow patients to do the work of the physician, enabling comprehensive remote monitoring. Telemedicine simultaneously necessitates more AI to increase diagnostic accuracy and monitoring capacities while providing the data for machine learning algorithms to identify patterns to make the correct diagnoses and interventions faster. The academic and business community could not have predicted the SARS-CoV-2, and the pressure is put on healthcare to become virtual. Any expansion in the scope of telemedicine sits on the innovations that will make the tricorder. As remote care makes its way to the forefront of healthcare, it brings the tricorder with it.

Rapidly advancing sensor technology is becoming integrated into the lives of physicians and consumers and dramatically changing research and healthcare. Along with the development of the tricorder comes diagnostic AI. Some physicians currently use medical AI for treatment and diagnostic testing, called AI or algorithm medicine, but only a small fraction do so routinely. It's often applied to generating adverse effect warnings for prescribing multidrug combinations. AI medicine will help pinpoint a diagnosis or develop a treatment plan in the future. Research in this area has been encouraging as algorithms have been developed that outcompete physicians in finding cancer, predicting heart attacks, spotting other red flags, and notifying the physician. All of these are done remotely without the patient waiting to feel sick to go to an emergency room.

The more serious a medical problem is, the more unreliable a computer's diagnosis becomes. Computers that create a trusted diagnosis remain far out of reach, but machine learning algorithms and AI can increasingly be trusted to solve specific problems. Physicians paired with computer AI diagnose patients correctly almost every time. The algorithm medicine of the tricorder is the future of healthcare, but it will not replace physicians yet. Aside from use by physicians and consumers, other applications of medical tricorder-based technologies involve the use of large-sized medical devices in kiosks at the entrances of hospitals. With time and technological advancements in miniaturization, tricorders may also lend themselves to technologies deployable in crisis zones such as refugee camps and areas plagued by conflict or stricken with natural disasters.

For a long time now, too few physicians have had to treat too many patients, which is only getting worse. In 2010, the AAMC predicted the United States would have a shortage of 90,000 physicians by 2022; by 2017, it had already reached 96,000 and is projected to grow to 189,000 by 2033. This shortage makes for physician burnout and higher patient costs. More importantly, it the lack of physicians increases mortality. If counties with fewer than one doctor per 3,500 residents had one for every 1,500 residents, over 9,000 fewer people would die per year, and the average life expectancy would increase by five years.

That's just in the U.S.. Globally, a staggering four billion people lack access to healthcare. This burden falls heaviest on rural populations and the urban poor. Tricorder technology will increasingly allow the patient to do the work of a physician, which will increase healthcare's reach and minimize the need to visit healthcare centers, and enhancing rural access. Medical tricorders promise faster diagnosis, intervention, and improved detection rates. By making physicians more productive, healthcare more efficient and less expensive as each innovation in tricorder technology will make healthcare affordable for more people.

Medical tricorder companies are conducting clinical trials of a smartphone application that records the sound of a user's cough. Cloud-based algorithms and databases of other coughs determine the likelihood that the user has several respiratory diseases. These trials focus on its ability to detect tuberculosis (TB), which, though it is curable, remains one of the top ten causes of death. In 2021,

15 million people fell ill with TB, and 1.8 million died. Most cases occur in the developing world due to poor access to healthcare, low detection rates, and the prevalence of HIV infection, which makes the likelihood of developing active TB roughly 27 times higher. The thirty countries with the highest TB burdens accounted for 87% of all cases. In short, it is a disease of poverty and a costly one. If this tricorder and its app pass clinical trials, it may be ready for deployment in the developing world by 2023. The new generation of medical tricorders will be tested for their ability to detect other respiratory illnesses. Considering the current COVID-19 pandemic, an smartphone app that could detect respiratory disease would have an incredible impact.

Soon, medical tricorder technology will be available and marketed for consumer use. In 2023, for instance, a comprehensive vital-sign-monitoring wearable will become available. Paired with an AI-powered smartphone application, it will measure and interpret far more physiological data than consumer wearables available today, monitoring mental and creative efficiency and advising when a user should take a break. Although many pieces of the tricorder have been developed or are in progress, they have yet to be put together in the final device. Various equipment needs to be miniaturized, and there needs to be more progress in portable computers so they can handle the information and data required for a complete picture of a patient's health. Also needed are more detailed diagnostics and less invasive testing. While the tricorder doesn't exist yet, the technology is closer than ever to allowing for its creation.

Risks and Challenges

The main challenges medical tricorders face are price, time to diagnose, and reliability. These are undoubtedly significant hurdles in tricorder development, but they will be solved over time. Though it's not possible to make an inexpensive personal tricorder today, the nature of the market continuously pursues lowering costs, accuracy, availability to a larger population, and constant monitoring of individuals' health. Medical tricorders, sensor technology, and AI medicine carry their ethical considerations with them. Both deal in big data and are subject to concerns over privacy and government and corporate access and use.

Currently, diagnostic algorithms are not reliable enough to make trusted judgments and, where implemented, remain only a clinical decision support system. Considering this, an AI tasked with alerting a physician to data from a continuously monitoring wearable would likely alert too often to be reasonably pursued each time, shifting liability to the physician, who would rather avoid it altogether. Many ethical concerns about the tricorder are posed by physicians themselves, who have been described as a conservative group in that regard. Some physicians do not feel confident that tricorders would allow patients access to their medical data. On the other hand, one can imagine a hypochondriac using tricorders as a method of health hypervigilance.

Some worry that consumer tricorders have the potential to encourage users to self-medicate or to make them less likely to make necessary hospital visits. A tricorder's AI must be carefully designed to neither promote underutilization nor overutilization of medical resources, given that both cause negative consequences. A company faces far more risk in suggesting a user seek medical attention too infrequently than too often, and considering the imprecision of diagnostic algorithms, avoiding the latter would be challenging. Many physicians do not trust patients with their medical data. Because of this, the physicians might be unwilling to adopt these new technologies.

Long before tricorder-based innovations find their way to those who lack access to healthcare, they will be used by insurance companies to examine customers, quantify their health, and evaluate their rates. While some innovations toward the tricorder lend themselves to humanitarian use, like those available as smartphone applications, many will have significant price tags. Governments and international organizations will need to actively work to bring tricorder technologies to the rural poor of the developed world and those in the developing world. Policymakers will have to be willing to regulate tricorders if their misuse threatens to overshadow their benefits.

Summary

Medical tricorders may help equalize and democratize healthcare regardless of location or economic status and help make healthcare more accessible and affordable, especially for the poor and those living in rural environments. As of 2021, over three billion people do not have access to healthcare. Even in the developed world, too few doctors and people are too spread out. There is a strong possibility that tricorders may also increase productivity and reduce the cost of healthcare. They may help maintain social distancing and combat infectious diseases like COVID-19 because individuals won't have to travel to hospitals and clinics as frequently.

By collecting unique and accurate remote data from medical tricorders, clinicians will have more information to use in decision making while streamlining workflow with automated monitoring. The medical tricorder can enable rapid intervention and save lives by using advanced data science techniques, algorithms, and pattern-identifying AI. By managing the total patient-to-provider experience, medical tricorders can reduce costs.

With access to personal medical tricorders, some mundane and straightforward tasks could be taken over by patients, freeing physicians to attend to more demanding problems. Although the currently available products are far from the ideal medical tricorder, they will be available as health technologies advance. The medical tricorder is coming and, in some ways, is already here. Tricorder-based technologies are increasingly integrated into healthcare, assisting physicians and expanding the scope of telemedicine. One can expect them to make physicians more productive and healthcare cheaper. Medical tricorder-based technologies will also make healthcare accessible to people who cannot access it today. With advances in sensor technology accelerating, consumers will be pleased to find highly advanced health-monitoring devices becoming increasingly available. Like any revolution, the tricorder faces some ethical concerns that need to be taken seriously. Its parent technologies, algorithms, sensors, and AI face unique challenges that they pass onto the tricorder. Everyone stands to gain from the development of the medical tricorder and the innovations that come with it.

Statistics and Trends

- The HeartCheck™ PEN handheld ECG device from CardioComm Solutions Inc. It is the only device of its kind already cleared by the FDA for consumer use. The pocket-sized PEN allows you to take heart readings within 30 seconds from anywhere, the moment symptoms appear.
- Dynosense's Dynosensor health scanner will soon be available. It's supposed to be able to measure up to 56 vitals in less than 60 seconds.
- The medical tricorder market is expected to grow at 5.4% from 2021-2027 to reach $7.1 billion by 2027.
- Statistics say 133 million individuals in the U.S. are affected by some form of chronic illness like cancer, diabetes, hypertension, heart diseases, stroke, mental illness, pulmonary conditions, etc. Currently, the economic impact of chronic illnesses is $3.8 trillion annually.
- As chronic diseases are increasing, so is the need to self-diagnose and monitor your conditions, medical tricorders make self-diagnosis easier and thus the high market growth expectation.
- Tricorder market trends are showing an upsurge in R&D in many bid companies like Qualcomm, Quantu, Scanadu, Cloud DX, etc. The total U.S. medical health R&D investment in 2017 was $182.3 billion and in 2020 has gone up to $294.2 billion.
- Based on end users, the medical tricorder market is bifurcated into hospitals, clinics, and others. In 2020, the hospital segment accounted for the majority of the market share. This is probably due to the greater number of

services available in the hospitals with its numerous helping staffs, and different departments as compared to clinics and others.

- Chronic Illness is a common condition throughout the world and especially in the U.S.. According to the centers for diseases control and prevention, 4 in 10 adults have 2 or more chronic diseases in 2021. Due to this, the need for self-diagnosis and monitoring equipment with the latest technology is high in demand.
- Since the onset of the pandemic, U.S. citizens are preferring to self-diagnose and monitor their diseases at home. This is likely to boost the medical devices market. Additionally, the recent 2-year U.S. excise tax moratorium on medical devices in 2021 is likely to decrease the prices of medical tricorders as well.
- The MedTech responsible for the innovations of tricorders is put in the center stage during the coronavirus pandemic. They are pressured with unparalleled demands for PPE kits, ventilators, diagnostic tests, and other critical medical supplies. Extraordinary efforts are being applied to ramp up manufacturing capabilities. MedTech leaders must go beyond their boundaries to explore solutions to minimize the supply needs by bringing tricorders to the market.

Chapter 11
Genome Sequencing and Editing

Contents

Introduction

On 26 June 2000, the U.S. and U.K. governments simultaneously announced the completion of the first draft of the entire human genome, the first map of the three billion base pairs that make up human DNA. The international project, led by scientists worldwide, aimed to provide high-quality sequencing data to help the scientific community understand human genetics, health, and disease. The final sequence was declared complete in 2003 as the culmination of more than ten years of effort.

This feat was built on previous research that had started much earlier. On 26 June 2000, the U.S. and U.K. governments simultaneously announced the completion of the first draft of the entire human genome, the first map of the three billion base pairs that make up human DNA. The international project, led by scientists worldwide, aimed to provide high-quality sequencing data to help the scientific community understand human genetics, health, and disease. The final sequence was declared complete in 2003 as the culmination of more than ten years of effort.

This feat was built on previous research that had started much earlier. Watson and Crick's research, which solved the problem of determining DNA's physical structure, came 50 years prior, in 1953. This discovery was shortly followed by years of research into accurately reading the sequence of the base pairs that comprise DNA and other genetic information. In the late 1970s, Frederick Sanger would sequence the first DNA genome and later develop a groundbreaking process that utilized chain termination to create DNA. A single nucleotide could be added at a time. This would later form the basis for what is commonly referred to as first-generation sequencing techniques. Future technologies would later emerge that could sequence multiple DNA sequences in parallel. Currently, the most advanced technologies sequence DNA without any amplification, unlike all previous techniques. The most promising future technologies in DNA sequencing are expected to be in nanopore sequencing, where voltage is measured across a membrane as an enzyme feeds through single-stranded DNA.

What is Genome Sequencing and Editing?

At the most basic level, genome sequencing is the process by which the order of the chemical bases that make up DNA are determined: adenine, thymine, guanine, and cytosine. This specific order of bases on DNA carries all genetic information for organisms critical to understanding almost all areas of healthcare. This information comprises the complete blueprint for the creation and development of all humans.

The most common accomplishment for genome sequencing is automated genome sequencing machines. In this process, scientists prepare DNA for sequencing by cutting it up and copying it many times over. Then, they add modified bases to the DNA that has the effect of making the new DNA section stop growing. Scientists can separate these four groups and label them with a fluorescent protein. They create groups of DNA, all ending in T with one color, A with one color, G with one color, and C with one color. Each one of these colors is noted which base it is connected to. The scientists employ the process of gel electrophoresis, where shorter pieces of DNA move faster than larger pieces of DNA. Electrophoresis takes advantage of DNA particles being partially negatively charged. Because of this, scientists can apply a current to the electrophoresis gel that the DNA particles are placed in, and the particles are forced through the gel by electrical attraction. By exciting each piece of DNA with a laser that reaches the end of the gel, they can then determine what base pair it is. The machine creates the genome by keeping track of the order in which each piece of DNA comes in. A marginally larger piece will reach the end later in time than a piece of DNA that is one unit smaller.

It is not necessary to sequence the entire genome. A variety of DNA sequencing is much more selective and focused that can still be informative for clinicians and patients. Examples include targeted sequencing, which is the sequencing of exons within a gene: single gene sequencing, which is the sequencing of only one gene and multi-gene panel sequencing, which is the sequencing of some but not all genes in the genome. All these methods can reveal information about inherited diseases. These more selective processes are used to look at specific areas and can significantly reduce the cost, time, and skill required to run a complete genome sequence. Clinicians will often employ these selective tests to look for specific abnormalities or sequences that would lead them to reach certain conclusions, but not so much information that it is unnecessarily specific in other areas that the clinician is familiar with.

Current advances are being made in next-generation sequencing. Next-generation sequencing refers to methods that can sequence segments of DNA in parallel. These systems save both money and time by using single steps on different pieces of DNA simultaneously. Three commercially available technologies that are referred to as next-generation sequencing follow. These systems are becoming more common in laboratories because of their ease of use, speed, and rapidly decreasing price as they are modified. Many research and R&D specialists will note that the perfect gene sequencing machine will be fast, cheap, easy, and portable. Next-generation sequencing solves almost all these issues except for ease of portability, a problem that is currently being studied and has produced promising working prototypes.

Illumina: DNA polymerase and modified bases with a terminator and fluorescent label are used. As DNA polymerase adds a base, it stops because of the terminator. A photo is taken to determine the base pair from fluorescence. Then, the terminator is removed along with the fluorescent label so that the next base can be added and photographed. This process is then repeated base by base until the read is complete.

Roche 454: Like Illumina, but instead are flooding beads with identical strands with a particular base. The binding of this base to the DNA via DNA polymerase will emit a light signal and let the scientist know the base pair at that location. These can then be recorded, and the sequence can be created after successive washing and applying single base pairs and DNA polymerase.

Ion Torrent Sequencing: This involves measuring the changes in pH by taking advantage of dNTP addition to DNA will decrease the pH by releasing ah + ion. One of the four types of dNTP is added (dATP, dGTP, dCTP, or dTTP), and the pH is detected. A PH shift will signal an addition of a base. The larger the shift will signal more bases being added. These shifts should be somewhat discrete as scientists are working on the release of protons, and the pH change should be clear in showing how many bases are added if there is a baseline control for pH change when a single base is added.

Gene editing is currently used for treating disease in both germline and somatic cells. Editing germline cells involves editing the DNA of sperm and eggs. This editing allows genomic changes in the offspring created by the combination of sperm and egg. On the other hand, DNA editing of somatic cells only affects the individuals who possess those cells since the patient's reproductive cells are not being edited. These individuals will not pass down these edited genomes to their offspring.

There have been a few cases where both germline and somatic therapies have been used. Usually, the editing or deletion of DNA is to cure a disease. Several methods can achieve this editing, but it is often done using CRISPR. With CRISPR, scientists can easily detect and edit specific portions of DNA. This process uses bacteria that can use a CRISPR array, acting as a guide, to cut DNA apart at certain places. Researchers can then use the cell's DNA repair processes to rebuild the DNA into an edited sequence. It is challenging to propose what gene editing will become in the future. Due to ethical and moral concerns, the scientific community has been held back by legislation from further research on the editing of human germline cells. There have been some documented procedures of somatic gene therapy, which are used only to alter specific tissues. Without allowed research, the field of human germline editing will not continue in any legal capacity. Research may be allowed in the distant future, which would likely propel gene-editing technology and capabilities. Without research and funding, scientists will unlikely to invest time and money into discovering new technologies to edit genes.

CRISPR and the Cas-9 protein accompanying it are already cheap, easy to use, and fast. CRISPR Cas-9 will remain the gold standard of gene-editing until there is a breakthrough in editing technology of nonhuman genomes: zebrafish, mice, and plants are very commonly edited species. Otherwise, governmental regulations change, and research on the gene-editing of humans becomes popular and possibly introduced to the clinical environment.

Uses and Applications of Genome Sequencing and Editing

Currently, there are various reasons for clinicians to administer or order genetic testing. One of the most popular uses for genome sequencing is to diagnose individuals that may have a hereditary disease. These individuals being tested are often fetuses. Because many hereditary diseases have been sequenced, clinicians can reorder genome sequencing for individuals they presume to have a certain disease, such as testing in prenatal cases. If a test comes back as positive, the clinician can be almost certain that the root cause of the symptoms a patient is experiencing has been found. This allows for diagnoses that are based upon symptoms and causes, the mutated or abnormal DNA, rather than symptoms alone. The results of these tests can provide information to the healthcare professional for treatment of symptoms and make informed decisions regarding family planning and lifestyle choices. Additionally, inherited diseases may present as similar based on symptoms. With genetic screening, medical professionals can discern the actual condition. Healthcare professionals continue to stress the need for patients to obtain a correct diagnosis from medical geneticists so that they can be properly diagnosed.

Individuals who are planning to have children may elect to have genetic testing done on their genome to uncover any mutations passed to offspring. This type of testing is very common and allows future parents a choice. After learning of a genetic disorder, parents may choose to have genetic tests performed on their fetus, in-vitro fertilization with germline cells containing known genetic information, or adoption. This "carrier screening," allows potential parents to make informed decisions before having a child.

Another common use for genome sequencing is for the treatment and specific typing of cancers. It is becoming more common that a cancer diagnosis is accompanied by a genetic test. Most cancers have different types, such as lung cancer or skin cancer. Many of these types are due to a specific difference in genome mutation. Armed with the genetic information contained inside of cancerous tumors, medical oncologists can make key decisions about how to effectively treat cancer. Usually, certain clinical solutions attack cancer in different ways. This may be how different drugs affect different proteins or how excision (the removal of a tumor) has different goals from chemotherapy. All of these solutions may only work for different individuals, however, matching the treatment to the patient is imperative. Pharmacogenomics has arisen as a popular study in how a patient's particular genome may lead to decisions about which pharmaceuticals a physician may employ, which can save money, time, and medical resources.

Legislation across nearly all major countries has all but stopped the current use of genome editing. Although the use of gene editing on germline cells was present in China, this experiment was a single instance and met with considerable public outrage because of questions regarding ethics. The lack of human gene editing is not because of a lack of technology. Scientists have proven they can quickly, cheaply, and easily edit the genes of other living organisms. The lack of concrete and international agreements on what is acceptable regarding the editing of the human gene has dissuaded almost all researchers because of the threatened consequences. It is, of course, hard to predict how a technology will be used in the future. There has been a wide range of proposed uses of genome sequencing that may occur, and it is more than probable that there are uses that have not been imagined. Still, the noting of predicted uses is fruitful.

First, research scientists and statisticians continue to stress the need for large population size data. Multiple major projects continue to fill immense databases with individuals' entire genomes along with the codes of other hereditary units that operate in humans, such as messenger RNA. As statisticians and research scientists continue to collect immense amounts of data regarding the human genome and diseases, it is expected that there is more to learn about the minutiae of how certain sequences can lead to the various processes of human life. Regarding oncology, liquid biopsy technology has been a very popular area of research that would allow diagnosis of tumors based on DNA segments present in the bloodstream and would also be able to type tumors by genetic sequence instead of common typing which typically is based upon abnormality and aggression.

Considering the movement of genome sequencing technologies into user-friendly devices; it is expected that the technology should break out of the research and clinical setting. The public has already seen the commercialization of genome sequencing in companies offering information about family origins, propensity for disease, or diagnoses of hereditary disease. It is expected that gene sequencing will continue to be used in more areas such as forensics, epidemiology, and other public health fields related to testing for bacterial or viral DNA, and possibly even used for the storage of data. These advances will be made possible by technological advancements currently focused on making genome sequencing cheaper, faster, and more portable. The advent of an easy-to-use handheld genome sequencing device will propel genome sequencing into future use.

The future of how human genome editing continues to be a hot topic of discussion for political activists, politicians, philosophers, and scientists alike. Because the science has been mastered, genome editing continues to be an ethical issue more than a technical issue. What is necessary is a clear path forward for human gene editing and concrete agreement on regulations for germline cell editing. With these regulations, scientists will be able to proceed without risk of retribution or breach of government law. Many individuals believe that genome editing will never occur because of how much press and consternation have been caused regarding the topic. Since public and special interest groups have found genome editing as an area where a strong opinion is held, it may be the case that the government will be unable to allow human genome editing to move forward.

Still, the editing of DNA and hereditary information continues. Research on the editing of human mitochondrial DNA differs from the actual human genome. This has been an area of research as the mitochondrial DNA can be changed to provide therapies for diseases linked to hereditary information. For years, scientists have been editing the genomes of non-human organisms for clinical use. By using CRISPR to inhibit the activity of certain genes then exposing cells to drugs, researchers can then expose these edited cells to certain pharmaceuticals. If they notice a cell that was once resistant to a drug, such as an antibacterial, become affected by the pharmaceutical, they can conclude that the inhibited gene is responsible for resistance. With this information, researchers can form medications to "workaround" these genes and attack bacteria resistant to most antibacterial.

Recent years have seen personalized medicine growth, which tailors interventions to individuals according to their genetic makeup. On the other hand, the advent of new genomic sequencing technologies, which empowered the high-speed analysis of multiple genes, radically changed how genetic testing may be utilized in medical care. Genomic medicine has already shown benefit in refining diagnoses and guiding therapeutic approaches. While some genetic testing procedures can be partially completed in the home by gathering samples, most individuals do not have a personal DNA sequencing machine. Because of the nature of DNA, this machine would essentially be a one-time use item for each individual.

The price, rarity, and lack of practical uses have kept genome sequencing in the clinical setting and laboratories. For an institution to see value in a sequencing machine, they must believe that they will be sequencing many different genomes. The techniques that are required to deal with DNA are also featured in the process that keeps sequencing in professional settings. The requirement for the preparation and proper handling of DNA is a necessity for the proper creation of a sequence. Because of these limiting factors, a complete redesign of any sequencing device would be necessary to be used in a location that is either remote, unsanitary, or at home.

As medicine becomes more focused on care outside the doctor's office, the process or parts of the process of gene sequencing may become ubiquitous in homes. The collection of samples may become easier, cheaper, and common. This may lead to samples being taken virtually anywhere: at work, at home, or a local drugstore. The growth of a large data collection bank for individuals' health would aggregate this collected data. Research of handheld DNA sequencing devices shows that these devices are currently not suitable for the sequencing of human DNA, but it is not unreasonable to believe they could be adapted. Microfluidic devices may produce visual signals such as color based on certain sequences being present or absent. These devices can provide real-time cheap testing for certain known gene mutations or specific high-interest sequences that may indicate disease or a propensity for disease.

Government restrictions have kept the mainstream editing of human germline cells from being commonplace in clinical practice, restricting gene editing to research facilities. There are recorded instances of individuals receiving somatic gene therapy for conditions such as cancer with varying degrees of success. Most of the gene-editing that is being done now to help human health is in the study and control of human disease. Many researchers edit the genes of model animals such as mice or chimps to study effects and differences in genes that may be like human genes. By learning how these genes operate in other species, the medical community may learn about human disease and its connection to certain segments of DNA.

Researchers seeking to control vectors of the disease may edit organisms such as bacteria, rats, or mosquitoes to control diseases that may be passed to humans. Famously, there has been a program that sought to exterminate a certain species of mosquito, the Aedes aegypti mosquito, that is responsible for spreading a variety of diseases including Zika, dengue fever, and yellow fever. Researchers were able to modify the genes of male mosquitoes so that when they mated with female mosquitoes there were no female offspring created (females are the mosquito that will bite) and the male offspring created will carry the same gene and slow the female Aedes aegypti population.

The Future of Genome Sequencing and Editing

Genome sequencing is a tool currently employed by a variety of physicians and researchers. Because DNA is the most basic hereditary unit, reading the individual sequence of base pairs on DNA can give clinical professionals some of the most detailed information about how individual cells are developing. Because of the recent advent of commercialized genome sequencing and reading, individuals have been given more control over when and how their genes are sequenced.

Genome sequencing for clinical and research use is substantial. Industry professionals use genome sequencing for a wide array of reasons. Sometimes the genomes being sequenced are not human. Research scientists interested in various research areas such as development, protein processes, bacterial drug resistance, phylogeny (the study of relationships between organisms due to evolution), and several others utilize gene sequencing. Because the reading of DNA can be used to understand historical relationships and current processes, it is a multifaceted tool. While one researcher may be interested in similar DNA segments that would signal that certain animals have a closer common ancestor, a different researcher may be interested in the same DNA segment because they want to understand how it affects the development or regulation of a specific protein or signaling molecule. The types of research that use genome sequencing are expansive and show how vital sequencing is as a tool in the innovation of the academic community.

Academic research often intersects with genome sequencing in the clinical setting. Since genome sequencing is still performed in laboratories, many individuals who perform sequencing tasks for patients also work with researchers. Because of the vast array of applications for genome sequencing, various clinicians may employ genome sequencing technology. Clinical geneticists, genetic counselors, and other healthcare positions often interact with genome sequencing technology and data. These professionals are specialized because of the amount of different genetic conditions. These specializations focus on the genetic disorder's medical area, such as cardiology.

Currently, most researchers have moved away from human genome editing because of ethical issues. Research facilities have access to the tools necessary to perform gene editing along with funding for explorative ventures that would not be affordable in a traditional clinical setting. Many of these researchers are still interested in modifying genetic information to help individuals. They have worked on non-human genomes and GMOs (genetically modified organisms) to make life easier. Examples of these organisms may be mosquitoes that are modified to control specific mosquito populations or genetically modified bacteria to produce human insulin for individuals who may have diabetes.

As the sequencing technologies progress, genome sequencing will become much more ubiquitous. The key to this is the movement of genome sequencing out of the laboratory. As soon as individuals can use a portable device to sequence genomes without extensive training quickly, the possibilities for applications are almost endless. Any profession that may require individuals to confirm their identity could greatly benefit from using DNA profiles as a replacement for other forms of identification. Additionally, professions that focus on identifying any organic material from trees to bacteria could be able to cross-check samples with a given DNA profile. DNA sequencing may also provide researchers with information about potential hazards. In the future, scientists may be able to identify viral genetic material that is very similar to known diseases such as COVID-19 or detect changes in animals' DNA that signal high radiation exposure.

It is hard to say who will be using genome editing in the future regarding human genes. There are, of course, expectations that there will be a continued modification of other organisms. Scientists' ability to genetically modify bacteria to create certain substances or have specific skills continues to push the limits of scientists. Additionally, the application of genetic modification of food has been an activity with both proponents and opponents. If it is understood that the science will become more refined and be able to amplify benefits while minimizing the cons, it is expected that genetic modification of most things such as food, animals, and bacteria, among others, will continue to be innovated upon. There always lies the grave question of ethics with human genome editing. Human gene editing could have significant impacts on the world and hereditary diseases. Still, this technology could also amplify socioeconomic differences that already exist and lead to more significant differences in accessibility to healthcare as it could quickly become a modified version of eugenics.

Risks and Challenges of DNA Sequencing and Editing

Many of the challenges of DNA sequencing are currently being researched. Current issues with DNA sequencing are the time it takes to sequence, the need for replication of the hereditary molecule before sequencing, accessibility, and data safety.

Ever since its inception, the issue of how fast a sequence could be generated has been a point of research. This challenge has led to many significant advancements in the sequencing field and continues to push research. The issue with long sequencing time is that it becomes resource intensive. Not only is it necessary for an individual to attend to the sequencing devices, but they can become "backups" in laboratories as researchers wait for DNA to be sequenced. Time is money and the longer sequencing times cost payers more money per DNA sequence.

The need for preprocessing procedures to be administered to DNA before sequencing has always been a feature of sequencing technologies. By amplifying the amount of genetic material, reading that material is easier because of the DNA sequence process. The issue with these techniques is that the preparatory procedure requires a certain amount of a sample to replicate accurately, and there may be errors. There is currently research into devices and procedures that do not require the replication of DNA to sequence and can sequence via a single piece of DNA. These techniques, however, are currently slow and expensive.

The nature of DNA sequencing leads to various serious questions about accessibility and data safety. First, everyone's DNA is relatively static (barring changes related to aging or disease). This fact may keep DNA testing devices in a clinical setting because it may not be reasonable for individuals to own a sequencing device if it is a one-time procedure, provided the entire genome is sequenced. Additionally, individuals have already become concerned about what it may mean for certain groups to have information about them based on their DNA. Suppose a corporation, insurance agency, or employer obtains access to an individual's genome sequence. In that case, this may lead to these groups making specific decisions regarding the patient's healthcare, behavior, or other choices that may be detrimental to patients.

It is not unreasonable to picture a scenario where a patient's health insurance premium rises exponentially because the insurance agency is now aware that the patient is much more likely than the average individual to develop a serious and possibly fatal disease such as brain cancer. Because of this, there may be a social pushback from individuals who should be sequenced because of issues regarding their data and propensity for sickness.

The challenges with DNA editing start with the ethical questions of editing humans, a very serious and controversial matter. The possible control over every factor of how an individual could develop brings into question accessibility, forced evolution, unknown evolutionary consequences, and how far DNA editing should go. These are questions with valid arguments for both sides.

Some may argue that DNA editing should only be used to change genes that will cause life-threatening diseases. This argument finds fallacy when we recognize that every individual will eventually die, many from disease. Additionally, there would have to be stringent policing and legislation to keep medical professionals from changing genes that have been found to correlate with certain levels of intelligence.

Additionally, DNA editing for only cosmetic purposes discusses the reality that individuals that look a certain way are treated differently. It is a heavily researched topic of correlation between height and how successful individuals are likely to be. Issues like this will undoubtedly lead to inequality if there is a price for DNA editing.

Finally, it must be recognized that any DNA editing changes cannot be easily "undone." If an edited animal or human can reproduce normally, it only takes a single instance of germline editing to forever change the traits passed down in that family. This would allow individuals to be able to essentially ensure that more favorable traits will exist for generations after the first editing with minimal or no medical intervention.

Summary

The rapid increase in population age, accelerating healthcare costs, and the growing burden of chronic disease present significant challenges to health systems worldwide. The U.S. government has recognized this issue. Such tests have potential. Physicians, parents, and caregivers can learn valuable information about drug sensitivity, multifactorial or monogenic medical conditions, and even family history. Despite some being difficult to understand, some tests analyze practical calls to action. For example, it shows that an individual should have a higher intake of vitamins A and E and iron and no lactose, gluten, or alcohol intolerance. It also reveals conditions to which one may be at risk, informative to take preventive actions.

Genomic information can help clinicians decide treatment strategies by classifying a tumor according to its mutations and corresponding drug sensitivities. In some cases, patients have been spared costly and complicated procedures, such as bone marrow transplants, based on a molecular diagnosis. Cancer treatment is also set to benefit from genomic information to predict how an individual will respond to drugs (known as pharmacogenomics) and inform prescription of the appropriate medication or dosage. Pharmacogenomic applications extend into many clinical practice areas, for example, in prescribing drugs such as antidepressants, analgesics, and anticoagulants.

Genomic information is expected to dramatically change pharmaceutical testing and use through disease stratification in the longer term. New research on molecular pathways underlying health and disease will continue to further drug development and design. Researchers are using genomic data to create new therapeutic applications for existing drugs (repositioning) with significant cost savings and better select individuals for clinical trials to find uses for drugs that failed earlier (rescue and repurposing). Better targeting of existing drug use avoids inefficient and risky therapy. It can provide savings for the healthcare system and the economy at large.

Recent years have seen personalized medicine growth, which tailors interventions to individuals according to their genetic makeup. On the other hand, the advent of new genomic sequencing technologies, which empower the high-speed analysis of multiple genes, radically changes how genetic testing may be utilized in medical care. Genomic medicine has already shown benefits in refining diagnoses and guiding therapeutic approaches such as cancer.

Statistics and Trends

- As of 2021, more than 40 million people have had their genomes sequenced. This remarkable progress has brought with it issues of data sharing, privacy, and inequality.
- DNA Sequencing market size will reach $25.55 Billion by 2028. Technological advancements in DNA sequencing, improvement in healthcare infrastructure and research facilities, and increasing investments in R&D activities are key factors fueling market growth.
- Fast, large-scale, low-cost DNA sequencing has propelled genomics into mainstream medicine, driving a revolutionary shift toward precision medicine.
- By sequencing individual genomes researchers can uncover large amounts of information concerning all aspects of that individual's physiology, from their susceptibility to certain diseases to the way they respond to specific drugs.
- Many diseases, including cancers, are caused by alterations in our genes. Genomics can identify these alterations and search for them using an ever-growing number of genetic tests, many available online.
- Healthcare will move more toward prevention rather than cure and genomics will likely prove an important

enabler in understanding the particular healthcare steps an individual should or should not take.

- In the U.S. the Cancer Genome Atlas has mapped the key genomic changes in more than 30 types of cancer. Such databases could deliver a definitive diagnosis in seconds, and even recommend targeted treatments based on the DNA of both the patient and the disease
- Genetic sequencing of cancer tumors is helping not only to identify particular cancers but also to understand what causes them and what could cure them.
- In clinical trials, gene editing is becoming a fast, effective, and increasingly affordable treatment.
- With DNA sequencing heading below the $100 mark, by 2025 as many as two billion genomes could have been sequenced.
- One area personal genomics is particularly useful in, is pharmacogenomics. The genetic information from an individual can, in some cases, be used to select the most appropriate drug to prescribe to a patient. This helps doctors to ensure that the drug has the maximum effect while minimizing any potential side effects.
- Personal genomics can also be used to predict or confirm a genetic disease. By looking at an individual's genome it is possible to identify genetic variants that may increase the likelihood of an individual having a genetic disease later on in life.
- CRISPR/Cas9 is the most widely used genome editor and is a powerful tool for understanding gene function. Because CRISPR/Cas9 is an RNA-based system, it can be more efficiently and easily modified than the protein-

based approaches and allows for targeting of multiple sites.

- Genome editing is widely used in studies in a variety of organisms. For example, CRISPR is used to make "knockout" models of disease in a wide range of animals, enabling researchers to study the underlying genetic causes.
- Genome editing is also is being used to change genes in certain tissues or organs, facilitate the study of diseases by focusing on culprit genes, create cell models of disease such as in human pluripotent stem cells and inactivate viruses in pigs so that pig organs could potentially be used as a source of replacement organs for humans
- The National Institute of Health (NIH) supports human gene therapy research, including genome editing approaches in somatic cells, for a wide array of diseases and conditions with grants, contracts and targeted efforts, such as the Somatic Cell Genome Editing Program.
- Somatic cells are any cells not involved in human reproduction. This means that changes in somatic cells are not inherited by subsequent generations. CRISPR and other gene editing methods, especially ZFNs, are speeding gene therapy approaches to treat many human conditions.
- In 2014, the first clinical application of genome editing involved the use of ZFNs to make human cells resistant to HIV-1 by disrupting a gene required for the virus to infect cells. In 2017, a clinical trial testing ZFNs to correct Hunter syndrome (MPS II) was launched. Caused by an enzyme deficiency, Hunter syndrome can cause abnormalities in the skeleton, heart and respiratory system.

Chapter 12
New Drug Development

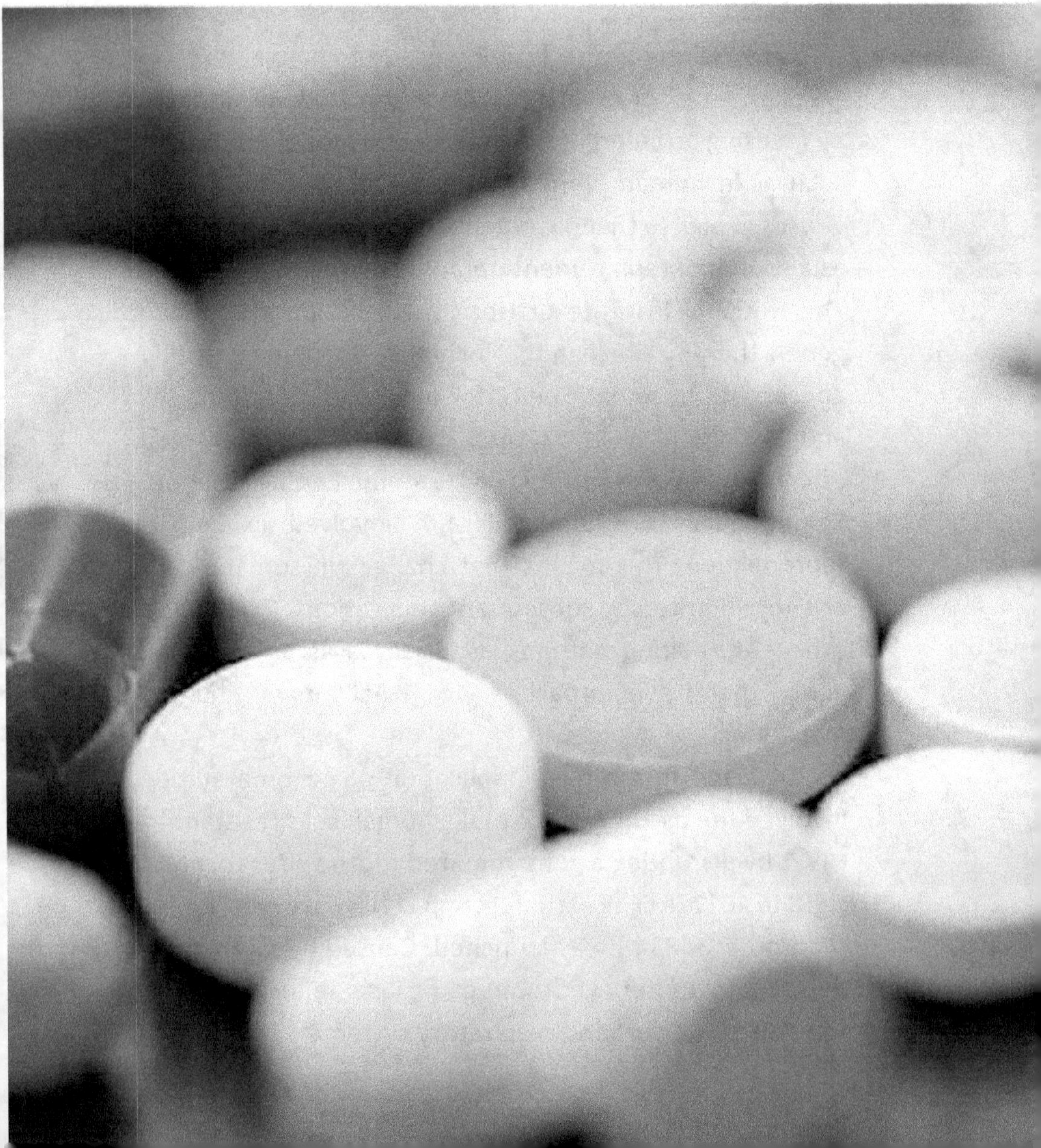

Contents

Introduction

Drug development has been around since the beginning of civilization. Drugs were used for healing and religious and spiritual purposes and administered by religious leaders. These drugs were often made from plants, animal materials, and minerals. The late 1800s was the beginning of drug development that followed scientific techniques. Now, drugs are discovered and manufactured in pharmaceutical plants at a much larger scale than in the past. The modern drug industry was born after World War I, and the relationship between drug discovery and scientific principles was established.

Modern drug discovery after World War I occurred over three main periods. The first was in the nineteenth century when mechanical chemists depended on chance to make their discoveries. The early twentieth century marked the beginning of the second period, which marked the finding of new drug structures; these aided in discovering antibiotics. Toward the end of the century, drug discovery quickly advanced due to molecular modeling, combinatorial chemistry, and automated high-throughput screening. Along with these new technologies, recombinant DNA technology allowed drugs to be developed for specific patients. Technological expansion and the "Omics" (a field of study in biological sciences such as genomics, transcriptomics, proteomics, or metabolomics.) This revolution has led to the third period occurring in the twenty-first century, with growth in biopharmaceutical drugs approved by the FDA (Federal Drug Administration) in the U.S. and EMEA (Europe, Middle East, and Africa) for therapeutic use.

Disruptive technologies and emerging trends such as robotics, artificial intelligence, 3D printing, precision medicine, and genetics will impact the manufacturing and distribution of pharmaceuticals. To prepare successfully for a better future in healthcare, the pharma industry is embracing new technologies and putting a greater focus on prevention and digital health.

What is New Drug Development?

After drug compounds are discovered, they are brought to market through drug development. This process has a few steps, such as preclinical research, which is done on microorganisms and animals, filing for regulatory status through an agency like the U.S. Food and Drug Administration (FDA) so human trials can start, and possibly gaining regulatory approval to market the drug. Drug development also comprises all the activities involved in transforming a compound from a drug candidate to a product approved for marketing by the appropriate regulatory authorities.

It can take anywhere from 5 to 15 years for a drug to be designed, developed, and approved for use in patients. Five crucial steps go into the drug development process of releasing a drug safely to the public: discovery and development, preclinical research, clinical research, FDA drug review, and FDA post-market drug safety monitoring. No medicinal drug can be sold unless the FDA has first approved it. The FDA only approves drugs that are proven to be safe and effective. If the benefits outweigh the risks, the medicine is usually approved for sale, though it can be withdrawn from the market by the FDA at any time in the future. Efficiency in drug development is critical for commercial success for two main reasons. The first is that development accounts for about two-thirds of the total research and development costs, so keeping these costs down is a priority for developers. If a drug fails late into testing, a lot of money has been wasted. The second reason is that speed in development is an essential factor in determining sales revenue, as time spent in development detracts from the period of patent protection once the drug goes to market. When a drug is patented, it cannot be produced and sold by other companies, so it is crucial that a patent last for as long as possible so generic competition cannot reduce revenue.

Uses and Applications of New Drug Development

The drug development process currently creates medicines that can be bought over the counter or prescribed explicitly by a physician. When used as prescribed by a doctor, these drugs can help treat many illnesses. One example is Attention-Deficit/Hyperactivity Disorder (ADHD) and narcolepsy being treated with stimulants. Central nervous system depressants can treat anxiety, panic, sleep disorders, and pain, coughing, and diarrhea are treated with opioids. However, the misuse of these medicines can lead to serious consequences, such as drug addiction or overdose. The medicinal use of drugs is to cure, halt, or prevent disease, ease symptoms, or help diagnose illnesses, and they have been used to save many lives. Most people think of medicinal drugs as taking the form of pills. Still, medicines can be delivered in many ways, such as swallowed liquids, drops put into ears or eyes, creams, gels, or ointments applied to the skin, inhalers, patches, tablets placed under the tongue and injections or intravenous medicines.

Biologics are a new type of drug that is becoming popular in recent years, even though in the past small-molecule drugs have reigned over the pharmaceutical industry. In 2020, 9 out of the 10 best-selling drugs worldwide were biologics. In oncology, the field of treating cancer, biologics meet needs that small molecules don't and are therefore used frequently. One such drug, trastuzumab (Herceptin), has been essential in many anticancer drug cocktails. Trastuzumab is classified as an antibody, but biologics also include gene-based therapies, cellular products, vaccines, blood, and other proteins. It is believed that biologics will be an essential component of future drugs. They are currently and will continue to have an important role in treating diseases like cancer, autoimmune diseases, and inheritable diseases.

Additionally, psychedelic drugs are taking popular culture by storm. From the psychedelic startup companies newly forming on Wall Street to a recent New York Times article that claims, "psychedelic drugs are closer to medicinal use," it seems that acid (LSD), mushrooms (psilocybin), ecstasy (MDMA), ayahuasca, dimethyltryptamine (DMT), and ketamine are making their way into the medical field of interest. To the extent that research has been allowed on drugs and medicines that aren't yet legal, there is evidence that psychedelic drugs can be used medicinally in the future. A JAMA Psychiatry 2021 study found that psilocybin-assisted therapy worked in creating antidepressant effects in patients with depression. A New England Journal of Medicine study also conducted in 2021 found that treating patients with moderate to severe depression with two doses of psilocybin did just as well, if not better at six weeks than patients who received daily doses of escitalopram (a common antidepressant medication). There is also great interest in the future use of psychedelic medicines in hospice and end-of-life care. They can help people overcome the fear of death, making dying a more meaningful experience.

Artificial intelligence (AI) is also being used in drug development. Its use (along with machine learning) will continue to grow over time, reducing the time to develop new drugs. Clinical trial models, such as virtual trials, will be innovated to reduce costs and hasten therapies on the path to marketing authorization. Overall, disruptive technologies and emerging trends such as robotics, artificial intelligence, 3D printing, precision medicine, and patient design will impact the manufacturing and distribution of pharmaceuticals. These technologies need to be embraced to improve the future of healthcare and put a greater focus on prevention and digital health. Pharmaceutical drugs are currently being used when someone has an existing disease to cure it. In the future, however, new drug developments (such as Biopharma) will allow for early detection, finding diseases before symptoms appear, and giving clues about the best way to treat each patient.

The pharmaceutical industry will continue moving from drugs to healthcare solutions, integrating other disciplines and technological products such as information technologies and medical devices. 3D printers are currently being used to create drug delivery systems. It is predicted that in 2050, 80% of medicine will be atomized, causing drugs and the pharmaceutical industry to play a different role. As the pharmaceutical industry moves away from mass production toward a more personalized model, 3D printing of drugs has the potential to revolutionize the market. The main benefit of 3D printing technology for personalized pharmaceuticals is producing small batches with carefully tailored dosages, shapes, sizes, and release characteristics. It also allows flavors to be incorporated into a pill without needing a film coating, masking chemical compounds' taste. 3D printers can be installed in pharmacies, hospitals, clinics, and remote locations, enabling on-demand production of drugs, particularly those with poor stability or cold chain storage requirements. 3D printing can significantly reduce costs, waste, and environmental burden for pharmaceutical companies as printers only deposit the exact amount of raw materials required.

It is also expected that individual genome sequences will be used to set up an informatics model with the ability to recreate body parts with that genome sequence; bioethics will have to catch up to follow this trend. Artificial intelligence will be one tool used to shift the field of medicine from treatment to prevention. We will no longer see drug prescriptions on paper; instead, individuals will have products delivered to their homes after a prescriber orders them online. Currently, drugs are either directly provided to a patient by a physician, prescribed and collected by a patient at a pharmacy, or provided at hospital emergency department visits. If a patient needs medical advice, their pharmacist will assist them through an application on their smartphone.

By 2030, it is predicted that the pharmaceutical industry will be driven by three levels of integration: products, services and data and technology. These three aspects will positively impact the patients' experience, as they will allow the adaptation of the medicines and treatments for each patient. Thus, research and development within the industry will be based on more accurate information. The idea is to develop a platform for clinical trials. These will include general trials in which several treatments are tested simultaneously, basket clinical trials where a drug is tested on patients with different types of cancer, and home clinical trials.

Moreover, the data will also help deliver much more than just medicine. These will allow early detection, find diseases before symptoms appear, and give clues about the best way to treat each patient. The industry needs data from other products and services besides the pharmaceutical industry to achieve this. This will involve collaboration between different actors in the health sector, as we have seen during the coronavirus crisis.

The Future of New Drug Development

More than 131 million people (66 percent of all adults in the U.S.) use prescription drugs. Utilization is particularly high for older people and those with chronic conditions. Most adults with one of five common chronic conditions (diabetes, heart disease, hypertension, arthritis, and cancer) use prescription drugs. For example, 89% of people with arthritis and 98% of people with diabetes use prescription drugs. People with these conditions fill many prescriptions annually and have significant prescription drug expenditures. Adults with diabetes fill about 4 times as many prescriptions and spend about 4 times as much on prescription drugs as the general population. High prescription drug use may also reflect the fact that people have multiple chronic conditions.

The proportion of people using prescription drugs and the number of prescriptions filled varies by demographic group. Prescription drug use is associated with age, gender, race and ethnicity, income, and health status. For example, prescription drug use increases with age. Three-quarters of those aged 50 to 64 use prescription drugs, compared to 91% of those aged 80 and older. The average number of prescriptions filled also increases with age, from 13 for those aged 50 to 64 to 22 for those aged 80 and older.

Women are generally more likely than men to use prescription drugs. The gap in prescription drug use between men and women is striking for younger populations. Some 40 percent of men and 66% of women aged 18 to 34 use prescription drugs. Use patterns converge as people get older, however. Furthermore, prescription drug expenditures are highest for people aged 65 and older. Drug expenditures are exceptionally high for the oldest adults. For example, average annual prescription drug expenditures for people aged 80 and older are almost 1.5 times higher than those aged 50 to 64.

The ultimate goal of drug development is to bring a new compound with proven therapeutic effect to the market. The transition from preclinical research to clinical stages marks a critical turning point as it nears the new medicinal product to the market. With the promise of marketing authorization, though far ahead in the road, hanging on the horizon, the approval of a clinical trial usually attracts investors and leads to a good rise in the company shares value. A robust and sustained pipeline of new and novel antimicrobial medicines is critical to ensure that innovations and interventions can keep pace with evolving pathogens that will arrive in the future.

There are many reasons why new drugs are necessary, such as the evolution of new diseases, the development of drug resistance, and our increasing understanding of health conditions allowing treatment of previously untreatable conditions. In some cases, it may not be a new drug required, but a previously known drug can be used for a new purpose. New drugs must be developed so that we can continue our chosen lifestyles and prevent the misery and death caused by diseases. Disease-causing vectors continue to evolve, throwing up new challenges, and in general, humans live longer, so they have more time to be exposed to diseases.

For many people, taking medication is a regular part of their daily routine, and these medicines are relied upon to treat disease and improve health. There are many benefits to using pharmaceutical drugs, such as lowering blood pressure, curing the infection, or relieving pain. While pharmaceutical drugs work faster to cure diseases and illnesses than herbal alternatives, they can also prevent other diseases and increase mortality rates. For example, regular use of aspirin is associated with longer survival rates among patients who mutated PIK3CA colorectal cancer. Patients who take regular aspirin doses to treat heart conditions had a 57% lower risk of death than those who did not consume aspirin. Besides pills and capsules, patients can also use vaccinations to help fight many conditions. Vaccinations treat illnesses like the flu, but they also produce antibodies that help prevent the body from contracting the disease again. Besides treating the flu, flu shots also help prevent heart disease and strokes.

Pharma has traditionally been attracted to large, profitable markets and developing drugs that are of "blockbuster status," usually at the expense of smaller markets with less reimbursement and less opportunity to drive return on investment. It is hard to imagine a shift focused on prevention, given the industry's appetite for large markets. However, with the catalytic effect of entirely new therapies, advances in technology, and the consumerization of health, it is expected that more targeted drugs will prevent disease and address the needs of specific groups of patients in other global markets. With the emergence of preventive medicine and precision medicine, valuable drugs will arise because of this diagnostic precision. Sequencing the human genome and the development of powerful and affordable DNA sequencing technologies has ushered in a new era of precision oncology. Patients are treated with customized therapies designed to target the specific mutations within their tumors. Companies that can develop drugs that target disease at the molecular level while minimizing off-target side effects and consider structural pharmacogenomics could transform the structure of the pharmaceutical industry and cure diseases with a significant level of precision.

Risks and Challenges

Several challenges come with implementing new drug developments into healthcare. Some of the main points include: drug development is a lengthy, complex, and costly process, entrenched with a high degree of uncertainty that a drug will succeed. For example, the unknown pathophysiology for many nervous system disorders makes target identification challenging. Animal models often cannot recapitulate an entire disorder or disease. Challenges related to the heterogeneity of the patient population might be alleviated with increased clinical phenotyping and endotyping. Greater emphasis on human data might lead to improved target identification and validation. There is a lack of validated diagnostic and therapeutic biomarkers to objectively detect and measure biological states. Drug development also faces the double challenge of increasing costs and increasing pressure on pricing. To avoid that lack of perceived commercial perspective will leave existing medical needs unmet, pharmaceutical companies and many other stakeholders are discussing ways to improve the efficiency of drug research and development.

The challenges are more extensive than ever, but the future of pharma looks promising. Biotech companies could lead the charge in scientific and business model innovation and be responsible for many of these shifts in pharma. And while consolidation of biotech by large pharma companies is likely to occur, a new class of biotech companies that rival large pharma will emerge. The pharmaceutical industry will reinvent itself and play a significant role in improving the health of billions of people around the world.

Summary

Drug discovery and development have a long history and date back to the early days of human civilization. In those ancient times, drugs were not just used for physical remedies but were also associated with religious and spiritual healing. Sages or religious leaders were often the administrators of drugs. The early drugs or folk medicines were derived mainly from plant products and supplemented by animal materials and minerals. Drug discovery and development started to follow scientific techniques in the late 1800s.

Drug development is the process of bringing a new pharmaceutical drug to the market once a lead compound has been identified through drug discovery. It includes pre-clinical research on microorganisms and animals, filing for regulatory status for an investigational new drug to initiate clinical trials on humans, and may include the step of obtaining regulatory approval with a new drug application to market the drug. Drug development also comprises all the activities involved in transforming a compound from a drug candidate to a product approved for marketing by the appropriate regulatory authorities. In the future, however, new drug developments will allow for early detection, finding diseases before symptoms appear, and giving clues about the best way to treat each patient. Drug development's ultimate goal is to quickly bring a new compound with proven therapeutic effect to the market. One of the tools that will be beneficial in the future is home clinical trials.

Several challenges come with implementing new drug developments into healthcare. Some of the main points include: drug development is a lengthy, complex, and costly process, entrenched with a high degree of uncertainty that a drug will succeed; the unknown pathophysiology for many nervous system disorders makes target identification challenging; animal models often cannot recapitulate an entire disorder or disease; challenges related to the heterogeneity of the patient population might be alleviated with increased clinical phenotyping and endotyping; greater emphasis on human data might lead to improved target identification and validation; there is a lack of validated diagnostic and therapeutic biomarkers to objectively detect and measure biological states.

Statistics and Trends

- The drug discovery market worldwide is on the rise. By 2025 the market is expected to be valued at $71 billion.
- The largest segment of the drug discovery market has been small molecule drug discovery. By 2025 the small molecule drug discovery market will be valued at some $48 billion.

- The top pharmaceutical companies based on their research and development spending are Roche, Johnson & Johnson and Novartis.
- Integrating AI into the drug-discovery phase can have a huge impact on the creation of safer and more effective drugs and the potential to drastically reduce the amount of time required to develop a new drug.
- Novel drugs are often innovative products that serve previously unmet medical needs or otherwise significantly help to advance patient treatments.
- In 2020, CDER approved 53 novel drugs, either as new molecular entities (NMEs) under New Drug Applications (NDAs), or as new therapeutic biologics under Biologics License Applications (BLAs).
- In 2020, 31 of CDER's 53 novel drug approvals, (58%) were approved to treat rare or "orphan" diseases that affect 200,000 or fewer Americans. Patients with rare diseases often have few or no drugs available to treat their conditions.
- According to the California Biomedical Research Association, it takes an average of 12 years for a drug to travel from the research lab to the patient. Only five in 5,000 of the drugs that begin preclinical testing ever make it to human testing and just one of these five is ever approved for human usage. Furthermore, on average, it will cost a company $359 million to develop a new drug from the research lab to the patient.

Chapter 13

A New Model for Health: The Neurobiopsychosocial Framework

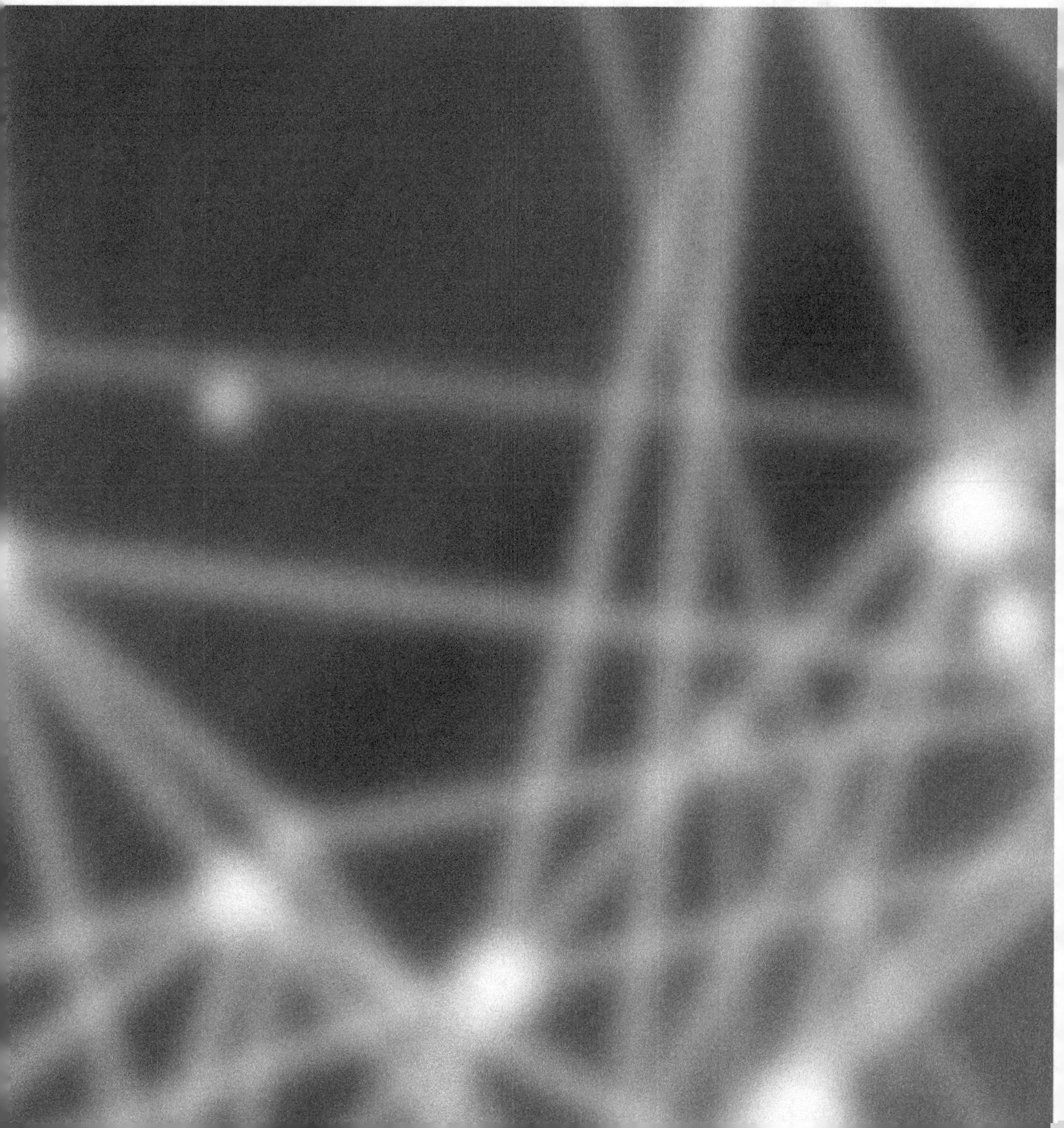

Contents

Introduction

Dr. David L. Priede introduced the neurobiopsychosocial interdisciplinary model on August 17, 2020, at BioLife Health Center. It adds to the existing biopsychosocial model, which acknowledges the impact of biological, psychological, and social factors on the state of one's overall health. The biological aspect identifies physiological alterations in overall health. The psychological part of the model reflects mood, personality, and behavior. The social element consists of environmental factors such as culture and socioeconomic status. The neurobiopsychosocial framework emphasizes the importance of the structure and functioning of the nervous system. The nervous system includes all structures and functions of the brain, spinal cord, and peripheral nervous system.

The neurobiopsychosocial framework aims to analyze further the effects of the most complex and least-understood organ in the human body: the brain. The functions of the nervous system are thought by many to overlap in the biological, psychological, and social aspects of one's health, which further stresses the importance of the neurological factor in this new framework. This new interdisciplinary model specifically analyzes how such factors play a role in health and illness.

The history of the neurobiopsychosocial model begins with two preceding theoretical models: the biomedical model and the biopsychosocial model. For over a century, the biomedical model of health has been considered the gold standard for diagnosing and treating patients. It has been used to understand the best treatment methods from a purely biological perspective. This framework relies on assessing measurable, concrete physiologic problems within a patient. The framework is based on the thought that all illnesses were sourced from measurable changes or alterations in one's body functioning. Utilizing this model involves physicians systematically assessing the patient and looking for somatic evidence of dysfunction. Because this model focuses so strongly on tangible evidence, it fails to address other factors that play a role in one's well-being. Psychiatrist George L. Engel challenged the model and offered a new way of understanding overall health. Engel believed that culture, natural behavior, and other psychological conditions significantly influenced the patient's health and how they coped with illness. Beginning in 1960, Engel began publishing literature criticizing the traditional medicine model, stating that it was not sufficient when treating patients. He produced a new model that he called the "biopsychosocial model" of health.

This model emphasized the importance of assessing psychological and societal influences that affected a patient's well-being. Utilizing this framework meant that the physician would look at variables such as socioeconomic status, religion, family and personal relationships support, patient perception of illness, self-esteem, and coping mechanisms and consider their importance when creating a plan of care for the patient. This new model initially received generous criticism from colleagues but became a fundamental model of health.

The neurobiopsychosocial model takes the same factors that Engel created in 1977 and tailors the model to include neurobiological alterations in one's health. Physicians who apply this model will look at the neurobiology of the patient for disorders such as trauma, brain injury, dementia, memory problems, depression, anxiety, headaches, and other chronic conditions in addition to biopsychological factors. The neurobiopsychosocial model reflects health development through the close interactions between neurological, biological, psychological, and social factors. This new model emphasizes the importance of investigating even further beyond the biopsychosocial model when examining a patient to provide a more inclusive and higher quality of care. With all these factors in mind, the neurobiopsychosocial model can be used today for an even more comprehensive and effective approach to health and wellness.

What is the Neurobiopsychosocial Framework?

The neurobiopsychosocial model can be understood by breaking down its predecessor, the biopsychosocial model, into three different key parts. The "bio" in the biopsychosocial model includes any somatic or biological factors impacting the patient's health. This factor relies on more concrete and measurable exams, such as a physician examining abnormal blood work in a patient with hyperthyroidism or evaluating an X-ray for a child complaining of arm pain. Genetics is also a vital component of the biological factor. Patients can have a genetic disposition towards developing certain conditions, such as Down syndrome, autism, attention deficit hyperactivity disorder (ADHD), bipolar disorder, major depression, schizophrenia, and others.

The psychological factor of the model examines the patient's psyche. The physician must consider variables such as the patient's internal feelings and perceptions of their illness. The physician must evaluate the patient's self-image and consider preexisting mental conditions that may be playing a part in exacerbating the current illness. The social aspect of the model includes societal influences on the patient and how these influences alter the patient's attitude towards disease and their capacity to manage it. This can consist of cultural and religious practices, family and friend dynamics, use of social media, socioeconomic status, and educational levels. Current stress factors in one's life also fall under this category. Events like job loss or divorce can contribute to the amount of stress an individual is experiencing. Higher levels of stress can, in turn, exacerbate or help to ignite illness. Combining these three factors can produce unique presentations for an illness in a patient. The different factors can exacerbate one another and cause diseases to be aggravated or subdued. For example, genetics can determine the susceptibility one has to an illness. Still, the psychological factors can play a part in whether the condition manifests in the patient, as with depression.

The neurobiopsychosocial model is a revised version of the biopsychosocial model that emphasizes the importance of neurobiology. This model encourages the exploration of the nervous system and its role in an individual's overall health condition. The brain is a complex organ. Much is still a mystery regarding its function and responses to the human experience. Numerous sub disciplines look further into animal and human behavior and the neural operations behind these behaviors. One example of this is neuroethology. Neuroethology is the study of instinctive human or animal behavior and the consciousness, thought, and higher-order activities in the brain that elicit these behaviors. External stimuli in the environment trigger various parts of the brain and evoke predictable or "innate" human behaviors and reactions. These occurrences can include contagious human emotion or the "fight or flight" phenomenon one experiences when exposed to danger. Another branch is biopsychology.

Biopsychology or behavioral neuroscience is the scientific study of the biology of behavior. This discipline looks at the biological basis of our behavior, thoughts, motivations, emotions, and moods and some of the deepest troubles we face as humans. This means assessing the brain's role in essential biological and psychological functions such as learning, thinking, sleeping, remembering, planning, etc. Disciplines such as these are the foundation for the neurobiopsychosocial model. Research into these disciplines can help physicians gain knowledge about the human brain and, in turn, can help them to assess, diagnose, and treat more effectively. Understanding the relationship between external stimuli and the natural human reaction can help researchers and physicians customize care plans for patients.

Applications of the Neurobiopsychosocial Model

The neurobiopsychosocial model was introduced to treat and prevent disease by taking a comprehensive approach to a patient's health while acknowledging the importance of the brain's influence on a patient's overall state of well-being. This framework encourages a patient-centered approach to health, encouraging the patient to express their needs and analyze their symptoms' perceptions and traditional assessment and utilization of technology. Using this framework, the physician can use various neurotechnologies to assess the patient while considering the impact of psychological and societal factors that the patient possesses regarding their symptoms. Each patient has a unique experience with their illness, requiring consideration of all influencing factors to have a complete picture of the individual's clinical situation.

The neurobiopsychosocial model can be used to manage several mental health conditions, pain disorders, and other chronic health conditions by utilizing neurotechnologies and understanding the relationship between the patient's symptoms and the internal and external factors that influence the course of the disease. Many patients who face chronic disorders have a variety of emotions and challenges that they face along with their condition. One example is a patient diagnosed with epilepsy. Epilepsy is a brain disorder where an individual experience repeated seizure activity. It is not well known what causes these seizures in all individuals. These seizures can have a profound effect on the quality of life of the individual experiencing them. When diagnosing a patient with epilepsy, the physician or provider can order and interpret a series of imaging and scans, such as an EEG or EMG, to identify the neurobiological factors marking epilepsy. The physician can then explore the patient's perception of their condition, their fears and anxieties about the condition, and the level of family and community support they have surrounding their condition. These factors can affect the need for different medications, the necessity of referral to counseling services, or the need for financial support with therapy. These all collectively determine the patient's ability to comply with treatment and remain well. By meeting these needs and ensuring that the patient can stay compliant with their course of treatment, medical emergencies and additional future comorbidities can potentially be avoided.

Chronic pain is a widespread issue afflicting more than 12% of individuals globally. Chronic pain can be challenging to manage and can cause significant distress in those who suffer from it. Many factors play into the perception and extent of one's pain. Because of this, it can be beneficial to treat an individual with chronic pain using the neurobiopsychosocial model of health. The neurobiology of the pain can potentially be assessed and diagnosed using forms of neurotechnology such as MRI, CT scan, or a Myelogram to visualize the source of the pain. At times, pain cannot be identified using typical scans, and diagnosis relies on patient-reported symptoms. Patients can have a differing array of symptoms based on several internal and external factors that affect how the pain is perceived. Psychological factors can include the patient's attitude towards the condition and any fears or anxieties the patient may have from the onset of the illness. Individuals may cope with their condition in different ways, requiring a tailored approach from the provider. Societal factors can play a part in the patient's ability or preference towards seeking care for their pain. Cultural views can affect the patient's decision to choose formal treatment for pain.

In contrast, socioeconomic status can affect the patient's ability to finance adequate treatment. Other clinical conditions, such as depression and anxiety, can stem from the patient's initial diagnosis of pain, which would need to be considered when creating a care plan. A thorough health interview and assessment of an individual with chronic pain can help identify any potential barriers and allow the provider to choose a plan of care appropriate for the patient's particular situation. Considering these factors optimizes health promotion and can increase the likelihood of treatment compliance for the patient.

Present and Future for the Neurobiopsychosocial Model

Medical professionals utilize the biopsychosocial model to understand the human mind and body concerning biological, psychological, and social factors. The establishment of the biopsychosocial model started to address and accommodate psychiatric disorders in clinical psychology. The principal foundation of this model is to understand health and illness better. This purpose still holds currently. The Neurobiopsychosocial model can be used in mainstream medicine to understand the complex interplay of multiple factors: neurology, biology, psychology, and the social element. This model can be applied to medical and physiological aspects and other fields such as health psychology, which examines similar influences of biology, psychology, and social factors on health and disease in the future.

Another application of the neurobiopsychosocial model that can be made is the perception of pain in neuroscience. Pain is a physiological response received by the brain to signal the sensing of a particular stimulus. For example, in a study done in 2021, there was a causative relationship between genetic and biopsychosocial factors in increased postoperative shoulder pain. This was partially done by examining pain-related fear of movement and depressive symptoms. Future studies like this are needed to comprehend how neurology correlates with our biopsychosocial model. By collectively combining four essential aspects of a patient's health—neurological, biological, psychological, and social—physicians and other medical professionals can utilize and reinvent medicine and use this model for improving the quality of life and preventative care of human health. The neurobiopsychosocial model was presented by Dr. Priede to primarily be used by physicians and other medical professionals in healthcare. Each area of the neurobiopsychosocial model is investigated and performed by a specialist in the area. Four area specialists use the neuro biopsychosocial model as a tool for treatment and prevention.

This model primarily benefits patients by providing the physician with a complete and comprehensive view of multiple areas of possible conditions affecting them. It considers patients' health from a complementary and integrative perspective, looking at the patient's health in all aspects of the word. The patient's treatment is broken down into neurological, biological, psychological, and social categories. The neurobiopsychosocial model's complementary and integrative outlook on healthcare helps physicians provide the most accurate representation of a patient's health. The neuro-psychosocial model is essential for proper treatment and differential healthcare. It is used for this purpose to benefit the patient's healthcare experience. As a result, the model is vital because it creates a healthier, more efficient dialogue between physician and patient.

Neurotechnology

Neurotechnology can be described as any type of technology that either helps one to assess the nervous system or technology that interacts directly with the nervous system. Neurotechnology has been in use in the medical field for decades, assisting physicians in screening for, diagnosing, and treating many diseases. As science has progressed, numerous new technologies have recently emerged to improve disease diagnostics accuracy and optimize health outcomes.

Imaging Techniques

Neuroimaging produces visualizations of the brain and nervous system so that structure and function can be assessed, and changes or abnormalities can be identified.

Magnetoencephalography (MEG) is a type of imaging that assesses the real-time neuronal activity in the brain. Several series of sensors termed SQUIDs (Superconducting Quantum Interference Devices) make up the inside of a helmet device that the patient wears during this test. These sensors cover much of the skull and work to provide an exceptionally high-resolution map of the brain that points out any active dysfunction. MEG can be used to diagnose disorders such as epilepsy and provide physicians with detailed information about the patient's cognitive function.

Magnetic Resonance Imaging (MRI) is a machine that performs 3D scanning and produces highly detailed imagery using a heavy-duty magnet. MRIs can tell much about the structure and functioning of the brain, identifying lesions and revealing blood flow patterns through a patient's brain. This technology is noninvasive and can be conducted with or without using contrast dye in the patient depending on the indication. There are several more specific types of MRIs that have various indications. Functional MRI (fMRI) looks specifically at the relationship of brain tissue functioning and the oxygen supply to the tissue. Researchers can determine specific areas of brain activity with specific stimuli by looking at the differing oxygenation levels in the brain during neuronal activation. This specific technology can provide copious amounts of knowledge for researchers in demonstrating the relationship between different landmarks in the brain. Another set of MRIs, termed Magnetic Resonance Venography (MRV) and Magnetic Resonance Angiography (MRA), specifically analyze out the vasculature system in the body or brain by using intravenous contrast dye to showcase blood flow in the given area. MRA imaging specifically looks at arterial blood flow, whereas MRV specifically looks at venous blood flow.

Computed Tomography (CT) is another type of imaging similar to the MRI but uses X-ray waves and computers to produce detailed visualizations of the selected body part. This type of imaging gives more detail than a traditional Xray machine, but less detail as compared to an MRI. CT scans can be utilized by neuroscientists to study structure, brain activation, and identify any abnormalities in structure. Intravenous (IV) contrast can also be used with CT scans to visualize any alterations in blood flow throughout the brain. This type of imaging is useful for detecting brain bleeds, aneurysms, past strokes, and traumatic brain injuries.

SPECT (Single Photon Emission Compute Tomography) is a nuclear imaging scan that integrates computed tomography (CT) and a radioactive tracer. The tracer is what allows doctors to see how blood flows to tissues and organs. Before the SPECT scan, a tracer is injected into your bloodstream. The tracer is radiolabeled, meaning it emits gamma rays that can be detected by the CT scanner. The computer collects the information emitted by the gamma rays and displays it on the CT cross-sections. These cross-sections can be added back together to form a 3D image of your brain.

Positron Emission Tomography (PET) is a nuclear imaging technology that utilizes positron emission markers to evaluate biochemical operations of cells. PET scans often require that the patient take a radioactive tracer intravenously prior to the scan. This marker will travel through the cells and scientists can visualize abnormal metabolism of glucose within the tracer, marking cellular dysfunction. This is helpful in identifying cancers, tumors, and subtle changes within the tissues that can often be identified as the first signs of diseases such as Alzheimer's.

Cranial Surface Measurements

Cranial surface measurements are non-invasive methods of measuring the neuronal activity in the brain and displaying live measurements of this activity for researchers and physicians to interpret and diagnose.

Electroencephalography (EEG) is a method of measuring electrical brainwave activity. Electrodes are placed in various areas of the patient's head and hooked up to a monitor where continuous waves can be read. EEG waves can indicate abnormalities in brain function, such as hyperactivity or lack of activity e.g. comatose states. This tool can be used intermittently or continuously to catch brief episodes of abnormalities, such as those who experience seizures.

Magnetoencephalography (MEG) is another method of measurement that complements the EEG. MEGs utilize helmets containing SQUID sensors and can detect the small magnetic fields generated by neuronal activity. MEGs can be considered beneficial over EEGs because the measurements are more precise and can give scientists a more in-depth picture of the relationship between certain stimuli and brain activity.

Transcranial Stimulation

There are multiple types of transcranial stimulation therapies currently being used to treat several clinical disorders with relatively low side effects and can be used as standalone or adjunctive therapy. The exact science is not fully understood with many of these therapies. Still, research is continuously underway to better understand these therapies and their application to improving quality of life.

Transcranial Magnetic Stimulation (TMS) is a type of therapy involving electromagnetic coils to stimulate the brain. Patients receive a series of "pulses" over the course of a 40-minute treatment that activates specific areas of the brain. This treatment is primarily indicated for treatment-resistant depression. It has been found in depression that certain areas in the brain exhibit hypoactivity. This therapy is thought to treat depression by stimulating and activating the brain areas that are involved with mood. Treatments happen periodically over the course of several weeks.

Cranial Electrotherapy Stimulation (CES) is another type of non-invasive therapy that can treat various mood disorders, including depression, anxiety, PTSD, and insomnia. This form of treatment has been studied for decades and is considered a low-risk adjunct treatment for these conditions. When receiving CES, the patient has a pair of electrodes placed on the skull or earlobes. Alternating currents are delivered through electrodes during the therapy session. Patients will continue to receive this therapy regularly for days or weeks until results are achieved. The exact mechanism of action for CES is unknown. Still, significant research on this therapy has deemed it a safe and effective treatment. This therapy is available to be performed by a licensed provider or can be purchased commercially for home use.

Transcranial Direct Current Stimulation (tDCS) is a type of neurostimulation that delivers low, constant brain stimulation using electrodes placed on the scalp. This therapy is still considered experimental and not completely understood. Still, studies are underway to help researchers understand its mechanism of action and potential applications for human treatment. Current research on tDCS suggests that this therapy can be valuable in treating chronic pain, mood disorders, and Parkinson's disease. There is also some evidence that this therapy may amplify cognitive performance in some individuals. Presently, this form of therapy does not have FDA approval.

Low Field Magnetic Stimulation is a potential new type of therapy for the treatment of depression. This therapy utilizes electromagnetic pulses and applies them to the patient for relatively quick treatment of depression. This therapy is currently being studied at NcLean Hospital, a teaching hospital affiliated with Harvard University. The therapy is also under testing for several other clinical disorders such as PTSD and anxiety.

Brain Implant Technologies

Brain implants, or neural implants, are technological devices that connect directly to the brain. The implants are placed on the brain's surface or attached to the brain's cortex. The general intent of brain implants and the focus of current research is creating a biomedical prosthesis bypassing areas in the brain that have become dysfunctional after a stroke or other head injuries. Some brain implants call for creating interfaces between the brain's neural systems and computer chips. This work is part of a broader field called brain-computer interfaces.

Neurological Devices are regarded as technologies that are attached directly to the brain and interact with the brain to either record or intervene in the individual's brain activity. Intervention on the brain via electrodes can help treat certain conditions such as depression, epilepsy, or Parkinson's. Deep brain stimulation involves placing electrodes within an individual's brain to stimulate brain cells.

Neuromodulation is the integration of neurological implants with neurochemistry. Neuromodulation is a newer technology that has been shown to have profound effects on numerous medical conditions spanning from treating chronic pain.

Cell Therapy

Stem cells in the brain are being researched to find uses for the brain, which recently have been found in a few areas. Many studies are being done to determine if this form of therapy could be used on a large scale. Experiments have successfully used stem cells in the brains of children who suffered from injuries in gestation and older adults with degenerative diseases to induce the brain to produce new cells and make more connections between neurons.

Pharmaceuticals

Pharmaceuticals play a vital role in maintaining stable brain chemistry and are the most used neurotechnology by the general public and medicine. Drugs like sertraline, methylphenidate, and zolpidem act as chemical modulators in the brain. They allow for normal activity in many people whose brains cannot act normally under physiological conditions. While pharmaceuticals are usually not mentioned in neurotechnology and have their own field, the role of pharmaceuticals is perhaps the most far-reaching and commonplace in modern society. The movement of magnetic particles to targeted brain regions for drug delivery is an emerging field of study and causes no detectable circuit damage.

The Future of Neurotechnologies

The future of neurotechnologies lies in how they are fundamentally applied and not so much in what new versions will be developed. Current technologies give a large amount of insight into the mind and how the brain functions, but further research is still needed to demonstrate the more applied functions of these technologies.

rtfMRI Neurofeedback (NF) delivered via real-time functional magnetic resonance imaging) is being researched as a method for pain therapy. Studies have shown a significant improvement in the way people perceive pain if they are made aware of how their brain functions while in pain. In addition, physicians can help patients with chronic pain decrease their symptoms by providing biomechanical feedback used to enhance both the learning and performance of skilled actions of the type used in sports tasks. Despite the obvious potential of biomechanical feedback to facilitate skill learning and performance, little is yet known, on how movement skills are controlled and learned.

This new type feedback is a new development in pain therapy. Functional MRI is also being considered for several more practical uses outside the clinic. TMS is being used in various potential treatments for patients with personality disorders, epilepsy, PTSD, migraine, and other brain-firing disorders but has been found to have varying clinical success for each condition. The result of such research would be to develop a method to alter the brain's perception and firing and train patients' brains to rewire permanently under inhibiting conditions. In addition, PET scans are 93% accurate in detecting Alzheimer's disease nearly 3 years before conventional diagnosis, indicating that PET scanning is becoming more useful in both the laboratory and the clinic.

Stem cell technologies are always salient in the minds of the general public and scientists because of their significant potential. Recent advances in stem cell research have allowed researchers to ethically pursue studies in nearly every facet, including the brain. Research has shown that most of the brain does not regenerate. It is typically a challenging environment to foster regeneration. Still, portions of the brain have regenerative capabilities (specifically the hippocampus and the olfactory bulbs). Much of the research in central nervous system regeneration is on overcoming this poor regenerative quality of the brain. It is important to note that there are therapies that improve cognition and increase the number of neural pathways, but this does not mean a proliferation of neural cells in the brain. Instead, it is called a plastic rewiring of the brain (plastic because it indicates malleability). It is considered a vital part of growth. Nevertheless, many problems in patients stem from the death of neurons in the brain, and researchers in the field are striving to produce technologies that enable regeneration in patients with stroke, Parkinson's disease, severe trauma, and Alzheimer's disease, as well as many others. While still in fledgling stages of development, researchers have recently begun making awe-inspiring progress in attempting to treat these diseases.

Researchers have recently successfully produced dopaminergic neurons for transplant in patients with Parkinson's disease, hoping that they will be able to move again with a steadier supply of dopamine. Many researchers are building scaffolds that could be transplanted into a patient with spinal cord trauma to present an environment that promotes the growth of axons (portions of the cell attributed to the transmission of electrical signals) so that patients unable to move or feel might be able to do so again. The potentials are wide-ranging, but it is important to note that many of these therapies are still in the laboratory phase and are slowly being adopted in the clinic. Some scientists remain skeptical about the development of the field and warn that there is a much larger chance that electrical prostheses will be developed to solve clinical problems such as hearing loss or paralysis before cell therapy is used in a clinic.

Novel drug delivery systems are being researched to improve the lives of those who struggle with brain disorders that might not be treated with stem cells, modulation, or rehabilitation. Pharmaceuticals play a vital role in society. The brain has a very selective barrier that prevents some drugs from going from the blood to the brain. Some diseases of the brain, such as meningitis, require doctors to directly inject medicine into the spinal cord because the drug cannot cross the blood-brain barrier. Research is being conducted to investigate new methods of targeting the brain using the blood supply, as it is much easier to inject into the blood than the spine. New technologies such as nanotechnology are being researched for selective drug delivery, but these technologies have problems as with any other. One of the major setbacks is that when a particle is too large, the patient's liver will take up the particle and degrade it for excretion, but if the particle is too small, there will not be enough drug in the particle to take effect. In addition, the size of the capillary pore is important because too large a particle might not fit or even plug up the hole, preventing the adequate supply of the drug to the brain. Other research is involved in integrating a protein device between the layers to create a free-flowing gate that is unimpeded by the body's limitations.

Another direction is receptor-mediated transport, where receptors in the brain used to transport nutrients are manipulated to transport drugs across the blood-brain barrier. Some have even suggested that focused ultrasound opens the blood-brain barrier momentarily and allows free passage of chemicals into the brain. Ultimately the goal for drug delivery is to develop a method that maximizes the amount of drug in the loci with as little degraded in the bloodstream as possible.

Neuromodulation is a technology currently used for patients with movement disorders. However, research is presently being done to apply this technology to other disorders. Recently, a study was done on Deep Brain Stimulation (DBS) to improve depression with positive results, indicating that this technology might have potential as a therapy for multiple disorders in the brain. DBS is limited by its high cost, however, and in developing countries, the availability of DBS is very limited. A new version of DBS is under investigation and has evolved into the novel field of optogenetics.

Optogenetics combines deep brain stimulation with fiber optics and gene therapy. The fiber optic cables are designed to light up under electrical stimulation, and a protein would be added to a neuron via gene therapy to excite it under light stimuli. So by combining these three independent fields, a surgeon could excite a single and specific neuron to help treat a patient with some disorder. Neuromodulation offers a wide degree of therapy for many patients, but due to the nature of the disorders, it is currently used to treat its effects are often temporary. Future goals in the field hope to alleviate that problem by increasing the years of effect until DBS can be used for the remainder of the patient's life. Another use for neuromodulation would be in building neuro-interface prosthetic devices that would allow people with quadriplegia the ability to maneuver a cursor on a screen with their thoughts, thereby increasing their ability to interact with others around them. Understanding the motor cortex and understanding how the brain signals motion makes it possible to emulate this response on a computer screen.

Challenges

Some challenges that may arise when considering the neurobiopsychosocial model are increasing effectiveness in prevention, improving the quality of patient care, and reducing healthcare costs while improving results and detection. As aforementioned, the primary purpose of the neurobiopsychosocial model is for health treatment and prevention. Thus, the aim of this model induces possible benefits that challenge today's healthcare system regarding healthcare prevention.

One challenge is how the neurobiopsychosocial model is centered on well-being and prevention instead of simply on treatment. The attention to multiple areas of study—biological, psychological, social, and neurological—our given model considers is primarily responsible for its effectiveness in treatment and prevention. This differential perspective is vital in our healthcare system today, as many aspects of a patient's life play a role in their health, not just genetics as previously believed. Not only does this theoretical model aids physicians in understanding how to treat a disease, but it also increases the level of detection possible in its early stages to be able to prevent certain health conditions. Early detection of disease also generates better health results and lowers costs; if the disease can be diagnosed before symptoms arise, that will lower the costs of medications and other forms of treatment typically required after diagnosis. Therefore, increasing detection and prevention is an excellent benefit of the neurobiopsychosocial model before unseen complications develop into a disease.

The neurobiopsychosocial model is a simple, cost-free alternative while rekindling the population's trust in the healthcare system by initiating personalized healthcare dialogue between physician and patient lost in today's era. Furthermore, this dialogue reinvents the concept of equitable and accessible healthcare for all. It ensures the reinvestment in new technologies, such as tele-counseling, as one example. Overall, the neurobiopsychosocial model aims to improve the patient's quality of life and care while lowering costs by emphasizing detection and prevention rather than solely treatment.

Conclusion

The neurobiopsychosocial model is a medical representation divided into multiple categories: neurological, biological, psychological, and social. All of the factors come together to understand human health and wellness fully. The incorporation of neurology makes areas and functions of the brain a focus of the model. The biological factor looks at genetic and biochemical influences. The psychological aspect deals with personality, mood, and overall behavior. Lastly, the social factor analyzes environmental and socioeconomic factors. The neurobiopsychosocial model was created by Dr. David Priede to diagnose and treat all health conditions and is expected to be used in various health-related fields in mainstream medicine. However, the overall purpose of the model still holds in that its goal is to help treat and prevent disease.

The current and future applications of the neurobiopsychosocial model include the treatment and prevention of disease by creating complementary and integrative techniques used in medicine. Medical professionals could use this framework to provide their patients with therapeutic and preventative interventions. In the past, the biopsychosocial model helped in debunking mental health stigmas in the field of psychiatry. Currently, the model serves to understand health and illness as a whole and the most complex organ in the human body—the brain. In addition, the summation of all of the model's associated categories provides a more wholesome comprehension of an individual's brain health and its accompanying components relating to biology, psychology, and sociology. This will enhance the patient's quality of care with improvements in detection and healthcare outcomes and lower the costs associated with the interventions.

Overall, the neurobiopsychosocial model is a highly credible model used in all fields of medicine. Due to its ample evidence of playing off one another, the previously mentioned factors considerably understand mainstream medicine and play a crucial role in health and illness. The neurobiopsychosocial model examines the neurological, biological, psychological, and social factors to explain a patient's treatment from a complementary and integrative approach. Furthermore, it will be widely accepted because it shows a significant improvement in a new direction in healthcare and a better understanding of health and its integrative and complementary interrelationships.

Chapter 14
Challenges

The healthcare industry is on the verge of a new era characterized by a preventive and personalized approach rather than a prescriptive and volume-driven one. The connected world enabling the digital transformation of our lives and society is pervasive. People often view the radical transitions as dehumanizing and technology moving us further from each other, making relationships more distant and interactions impersonal. However, this doesn't hold up to scrutiny when considering the context of human history.

We've never been so connected to people and information, and we are becoming more engaged every day. We can stay in touch with family and friends more easily, share experiences even though distant, and share intimate ideas over smartphone videos even when sitting next to each other. Like many essential areas of our lives, the connected world's realization also transforms healthcare. These solutions have yet to evolve entirely because current offerings require time and regulatory approval before use. Proof of efficacy requires extensive clinical trials that are costly and time-consuming, which can discourage some manufacturers.

The best part is that all these data points connections are another sweeping change in managing health—for example, access to medical records. Traditionally, physicians and hospitals kept patients from accessing their medical records or, at best, making it inconvenient to access them. One reason is that, until recently, medical records were kept on paper. But considering the staggering 400,000 deaths reported each year in the U.S. linked to medical errors, inefficient medical record-keeping is far from just a privacy and access issue. Luckily, a positive trend is a rapid transition to electronic health records (EHRs). While it's a positive advancement that patients will soon have complete access to present and future health information, it could pose a problem, specifically for future consumers and producers of massive, personalized health data. Having too much data can lead to the same result as having too little.

One of the big new industries set to grow over the next two decades is subscription-based personal health management. Patients will digitally share all their health data with a medical service. This service will then monitor patient's health 24/7 and alert them about impending health issues, remind them when to take medications, offer early medical advice and prescriptions, facilitate a virtual physician's appointment, and even schedule a visit at a clinic or hospital when needed on the patient's behalf. These services will strive to make looking after one's health as effortless as possible, so patients do not have to become overwhelmed or discouraged.

This last point is significant for those recovering from a surgery or major injury, suffering from a chronic medical condition, eating disorders, or addiction issues. This constant health monitoring and feedback will act as a support service to help people stay on top of their health. Moreover, these services are likely to be paid for in part or in full by insurance companies, as they'll have a financial interest in keeping patients as healthy as possible for as long as possible. The chances are that these services may become owned entirely by insurance companies one day. Many stakeholders believe that for these future health technologies to change how to treat and diagnose health issues, they need to improve the way data is interpreted and then shared with healthcare professionals. For example, an advanced tracker that can detect heart problems may sound like a life-saving wearable. Still, if the data isn't easy to understand, sent to a physician, or adequately considered for future treatment, it won't be as helpful as it could be. It could just prove to be more confusing. Of course, health tech manufacturers are responsible for

Developing better systems to interpret data for patients and make it easily accessible and secure. But there's only so much that individuals can do with potentially complicated medical information. This is where physicians come in and why it's imperative that they understand these future technologies' potential and how to use, access, and interpret the data it collects. Although implementing new ways of tracking and diagnosing issues might seem like a costly undertaking, it certainly makes sense for both patients and medical professionals. Many physicians do not believe patients can be trusted with their medical data and are reluctant to give access to it. Physicians and the public will push to adopt new digital technologies in healthcare.

The healthcare industry faces the challenges of addressing ever-increasing patient expectations and lowering costs while still providing consistent product quality. These challenges must be addressed, driven by greater efficiency, pricing and exclusivity advantages, and the ability to satisfy previously unmet medical needs. Many healthcare companies realize that they must reinvent themselves to address this transformation. Challenges include new competitors and first-to-market pressure, ever-changing regulations, rising development costs and time, pricing pressure, the shift to outcome-based economic models, the management of partnerships, and the reinvention of business models. These new trends will help reshape the U.S. healthcare system from a reactive to a proactive service industry focused on preventing illness and injury. Due to the high cost of bringing a single new technology to market, healthcare companies have more pressure to maximize revenue while staying ahead of the competition. Considering that programs for innovative products are high risk/reward, many companies continue to focus their activities on developing first-in-class treatments. The most innovative among them is developing novel formulation strategies and delivery systems that vastly improve patient experience and financial constraints.

Epilogue

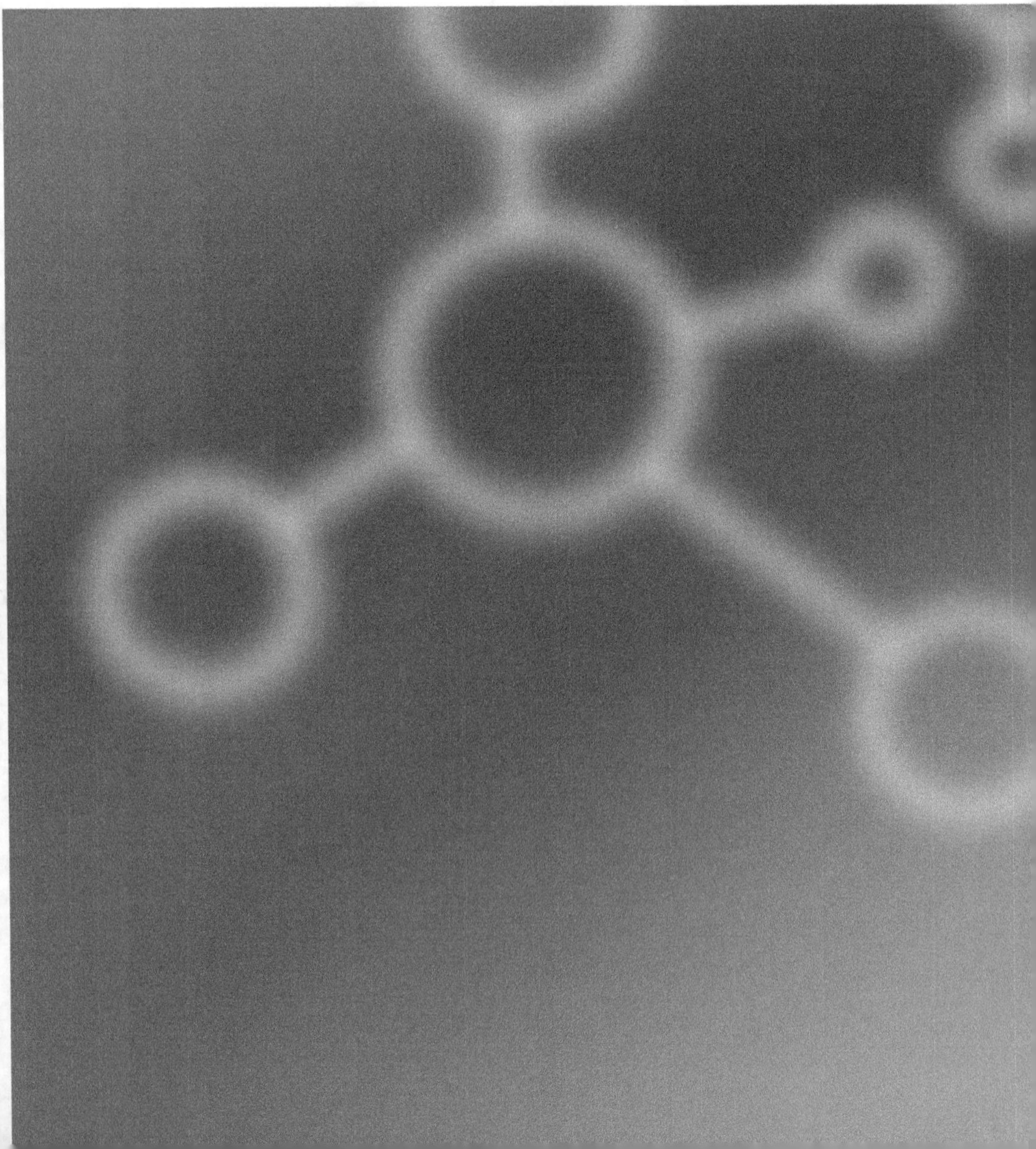

The new technologies being introduced in the coming eras of the medical field will not be here by tomorrow. With all of the risks, challenges, and obstacles new ideas must go through to be perfected, there is still plenty of work to be done. But there are already advancements and new technologies being used in the medical and scientific fields that were not there ten years ago. And with the help of these new technologies, more physicians, specialists, and clinicians can take on more significant volumes of work that would have been unprecedented with older technologies. Diagnoses and health monitoring will be faster, more accurate, and more convenient.

The biggest challenge the public may face when researching these new technologies is the impersonal nature seen at first glance. The world is quickly advancing in the digital age, and medicine follows. The entire process of visiting a doctor and receiving medical care is rapidly changing. How can we know if implementing these new changes and technologies will be more beneficial in the long run? Unfortunately, we can't say for sure, but research is key to understanding, and the new advancements also mean creating a more accessible and inclusive healthcare system.

With more focus on volume, there is a higher chance of more people being treated and more accurate diagnoses given to those who otherwise may not have gotten the proper treatment. In addition, there will be new ways that data will be managed in a way that hasn't been seen before. The new uses of data will provide a growing comprehensive means of eradicating error that is unfortunately commonplace today. Too often, we see patients being treated for an issue they don't have or not being treated at all for their problems because of the current technologies that form the basis for diagnosing and treating illness. New technologies remain beneficial because of their focus on removing errors. However, another central question is if doctors and clinicians can comprehend the new radical process of diagnosing, treating, and monitoring. As the public learns more about these technologies, doctors must know how to participate in these new objectives. If patients are the priority, finding the best effective treatment methods should also be a top priority.

We have discussed how new technologies and prototypes for these technologies have already been implemented through all these chapters. Advances in nanomedicine allow for noninvasive procedures to occur. Health trackers and wearables create sustainable forms of remote care that can even help prevent illness and disease. Even concepts such as 3D printing create new prototypical resources for mobility that are more cost-effective. However, changes need to be made before they go into the mainstream. This means radically changing the healthcare system so more people can be treated than previously. Today, standards in healthcare mean not everyone receives proper care. Many may not even be able to afford adequate treatment. Looking to the future of health, emerging technologies create a suitable answer for the medical field's issues. We must expect success and failure when promoting and researching new technologies.

However, maintaining hope in an emerging technology meant to better patients keep us from only looking at how things are working well now. We need to look at how things can be improved if we want to see any progress. Introducing emerging technologies allows new scientific and clinical research methods to be explored. If patients are to be the priority, we must continue looking to future technologies to see how they benefit patients and better help them than current methods do. With factors such as continuous health monitoring, remote nursing, and artificial intelligence diagnoses, patients can experience less demanding, costly, and invasive procedures and processes in the future.

Many more people now can hope to attain medical care they may not be able to have today. And the introduction of AI and other technologies limits the burden placed on nurses and doctors, eradicating human error and allowing more patients to be seen without doubling a workload. No matter what the medical fields face, new steps toward the future mean saving lives and treating patients for both major and minor issues. It also means we become more knowledgeable on how we plan to care for our health and how we can do that. As new emerging technologies are implemented, we enter the future of health, a future that does not let the obstacle we face get the best of us.

References

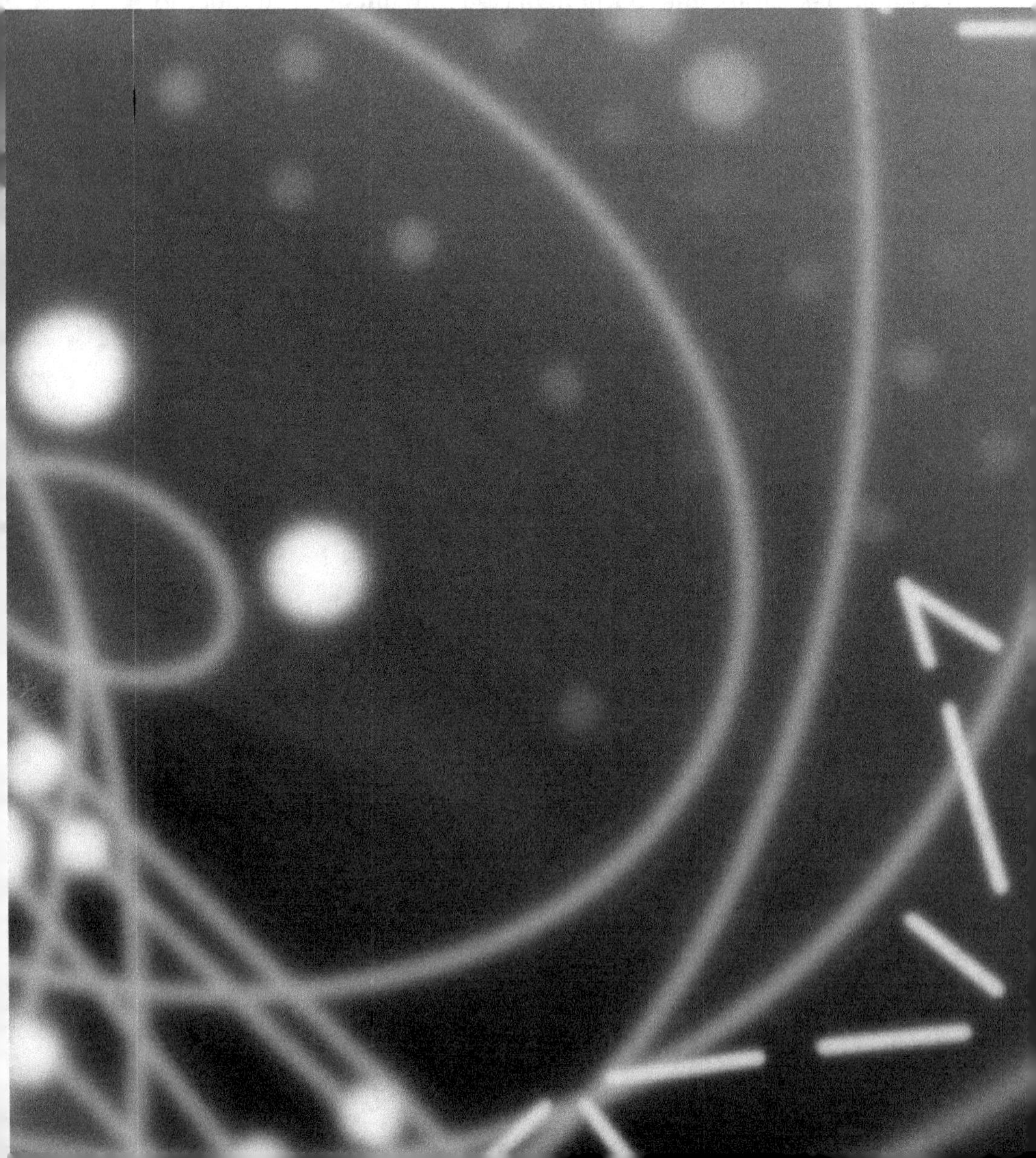

Chapter 2 - Virtual Healthcare

"History of Telemedicine & Telehealth: When Did It Start." (Nov. 2020) EVisit. evisit.com/resources/history-of-telemedicine/.

3 Ways to Humanize the Virtual Health Care Experience. (Jan 2020). https://hbr.org/2021/03/3-ways-to-humanize-the-virtual-health-care-experience

Benefits of Telemedicine | Johns Hopkins Medicine. (Nov. 2021). https://www.hopkinsmedicine.org/health/treatment-tests-and-therapies/benefits-of-telemedicine

Bhatia R.S., Chu C., Pang A., Tadrous M., Stamenova V., Cram P. Virtual care use before and during the COVID-19 pandemic: a repeated cross-sectional study. CMAJ Open. 2021;9(1):E107–E114.

Canadian Medical Association Virtual Care in Canada: Discussion Paper (2021). https://www.cma.ca/sites/default/files/pdf/News/Virtual_Care_discussionpaper_v2EN.pdf Accessed September 18, 2021.

Challenges in the Telehealth Industry | UIC Health Informatics. (2017). https://healthinformatics.uic.edu/blog/challenges-facing-the-telehealth-industry/

COVID-19 Survey: Doctors Like Telehealth and Want to Continue. (2019). https://mhealthintelligence.com/news/covid-19-survey-doctors-like-telehealth-and-want-to-continue-using-it

Fact Sheet: Telehealth | AHA. (September. 2020). https://www.aha.org/factsheet/telehealth

Gatto F., Khorrami K., Nista F., Corica G., Ferone D. Acromegaly management in a tertiary referral center after 1 year of the coronavirus 2019 pandemic: a double challenge. Endocr Pract. 2021;27(8):856–857.

Rubin R. COVID-19's crushing effects on medical practices, some of which might not survive. JAMA. 2020;324(4):321–323.

Telehealth. (Apr. 2020.). https://www.ama-assn.org/practice-management/digital/telehealth-s-post-pandemic-future-where-do-we-go-here

Telemedicine: Ultimate Guide - Everything You Need to Know. (January 2021). https://evisit.com/resources/what-is-telemedicine/

The Future of Virtual Care: How Combining Technologies Will Play (2019). https://www.himss.org/resources/future-virtual-care-how-combining-technologies-will-play-essential-role

The future of virtual health | Modern Healthcare. (2020). https://www.modernhealthcare.com/technology/future-virtual-health

Using Telehealth to Expand Access to Essential Health Services. (2019). https://www.cdc.gov/coronavirus/2019-ncov/hcp/telehealth.html

What is Virtual Health Care? (December 2010.). https://www.concorde.edu/about-us/blog/health-care-insights/health-care-awareness-virtual-care

Chapter 3 - Artificial Intelligence

Ahorsu, D. K., Lin, C.-Y., & Pakpour, A. H. (2020). The Association Between Health Status and Insomnia, Mental Health, and Preventive Behaviors: The Mediating Role of Fear of COVID-19. Gerontology and Geriatric Medicine. https://doi.org/10.1177/2333721420966081

AI, Automation, and the Future of Work: Ten Things to Solve for Briefing Note Prepared for the Tech4Good Summit, Organized by the French Presidency (June 2018). http://dln.jaipuria.ac.in:8080/jspui/bitstream/123456789/1335/1/MGI-Briefing-Note-AI-automation-and-the-future-of-work_June2018.pdf

Alexa, Siri, Cortana, and More: An Introduction to Voice Assistants. (2018). Medical Reference Services Quarterly. https://www.tandfonline.com/doi/abs/10.1080/02763869.2018.1404391

Allam, Z., Dey, G., & Jones, D. (2020). Artificial Intelligence (AI) Provided Early Detection of the Coronavirus (COVID-19) in China and Will Influence Future Urban Health Policy Internationally. AI, 1(2), 156–165. MDPI AG. https://doi.org/10.3390/ai1020009

Anderson, J., & Rainie, L. (2018, December 10). Artificial Intelligence and the Future of Humans. Pew Research Center: Internet, Science & Tech; https://www.pewresearch.org/internet/2018/12/10/artificial-intelligence-and-the-future-of-humans

Aniqa Mazhar. (2019, September 26). Evolution of Artificial Intelligence in Healthcare -. Scientiamag.org. https://scientiamag.org/evolution-of-artificial-intelligence-in-healthcare/

Application of Artificial Intelligence Methods to Pharmacy Data for Cancer Surveillance and Epidemiology Research: A Systematic Review | JCO Clinical Cancer Informatics. (2020). JCO Clinical Cancer Informatics. https://ascopubs.org/doi/full/10.1200/CCI.20.00101

Artificial Intelligence - CAR - Canadian Association of Radiologists. (2020, January 31). CAR - Canadian Association of Radiologists. https://car.ca/innovation/artificial-intelligence/

Artificial intelligence: threats and opportunities | News | European Parliament. (2020). Europa.eu. https://www.europarl.europa.eu/news/en/headlines/priorities/artificial-intelligence-in-the-eu/20200918STO87404/artificial-intelligence-threats-and-opportunities

Asadi, J., & Fariborz Tarokh. (2019). How The Artificial Intelligence is Helping to Cure: The Analytic Means of Health in Current Pandemic World. International Journal of Modern Engineering Technologies, 1(1). https://icdst.ir/OAJ/index.php/IJMET/article/view/22/49

Bajwa, M. N., Muta, K., Malik, M. I., Siddiqui, S. A., Braun, S. A., Homey, B., Dengel, A., & Ahmed, S. (2020). Computer-Aided Diagnosis of Skin Diseases Using Deep Neural Networks. Applied Sciences, 10(7), 2488. https://doi.org/10.3390/app10072488

Brown, Jennings. (July 25). IBM Watson Reportedly Recommended Cancer Treatments That Were "Unsafe and Incorrect." Gizmodo; Gizmodo. https://gizmodo.com/ibm-watson-reportedly-recommended-cancer-treatments-tha-1827868882

Davenport, T., & Ronanki, R. (2018). Artificial Intelligence for the Real World Don't start with moon shots. Harvard Business Review. https://www.kungfu.ai/wp-content/uploads/2019/01/R1801H-PDF-ENG.pdf

Gammon, Katharine. (2017, December 4). 5 Ways Artificial Intelligence Will Change the World by 2050 | USC Trojan Family Magazine. https://news.usc.edu/trojan-family/five-ways-ai-will-change-the-world-by-2050/

Gerke, S., Minssen, T., & Cohen, G. (2020). Ethical and legal challenges of artificial intelligence-driven healthcare. Artificial Intelligence in Healthcare, 295–336. https://doi.org/10.1016/b978-0-12-818438-7.00012-5

Google Health's Machine Learning System Diagnoses Breast Cancer Better Than Humans - BioMed Advances. (2020, January 6). BioMed Advances. https://biomedadvances.com/google-healths-machine-learning-system-diagnoses-breast-cancer-better-than-humans/

Hondt, C., De Winne, R., Ghysels, E., & Raymond, S. (2019). Artificial Intelligence Alter Egos: Who might benefit from robo-investing? Journal of Empirical Finance. https://dial.uclouvain.be/pr/boreal/object/boreal%3A238318/datastream/PDF_01/view

Institute of Medicine (US) Committee on Regional Health Data Networks, Donaldson, M. S., & Lohr, K. N. (2020). Confidentiality and Privacy of Personal Data. Nih.gov; National Academies Press (US). https://www.ncbi.nlm.nih.gov/books/NBK236546/

Marr Contributor, B. (2020). How Is AI Used In Education -- Real World Examples Of Today And A Peek Into The Future Enterprise & Cloud. http://gdac.uqam.ca/inf7470/IAetEducation/How%20Is%20AI%20Used%20In%20Education%20Real%20World%20Examples%20Of%20Today%20And%20A%20Peek%20Into%20The%20Future.pdf

Nadarzynski, T., Miles, O., Cowie, A., & Ridge, D. (2019). Acceptability of artificial intelligence (AI)-led chatbot services in healthcare: A mixed-methods study. PubMed. https://doi.org/10.1177/2055207619871808

Nasirian, F., Ahmadian, M., & Lee, O. K. D. (2017). AI-based voice assistant systems: Evaluating from the interaction and trust perspectives

Pianykh, O. S., Langs, G., Dewey, M., Enzmann, D. R., Herold, C. J., Schoenberg, S. O., & Brink, J. A. (2020). Continuous learning AI in radiology: implementation principles and early applications. Radiology, 297(1), 6-14

Quest, D. (2021). Demystifying AI in Healthcare: Historical Perspectives and Current Considerations. Physician Leadership. https://www.physicianleaders.org/news/demystifying-ai-in-healthcare-historical-perspectives-and-current-considerations

Select Committee on Artificial Intelligence Report of Session 2017-19 AI in the UK: ready, willing and able? (2018, April 16). House of Lords. https://publications.parliament.uk/pa/ld201719/ldselect/ldai/100/100.pdf

TD sees big role for AI in fraud detection, lending decisions - BNN Bloomberg. (2020, December 10). BNN. Bloomberg News. https://www.bnnbloomberg.ca/td-sees-big-role-for-ai-in-fraud-detection-lending-decisions-1.1534478

The AI Now Report The Social and Economic Implications of Artificial Intelligence Technologies in the Near-Term. (2016, September 22). AI Now. https://www.artificialintelligencenow.com/media/documents/AINowSummaryReport_3_RpmwKHu.pdf

The Future of Management in an AI World Redefining Purpose and Strategy in the Fourth Industrial Revolution Edited by Jordi Canals Franz Heukamp. (2020). IESE Business School University of Navarra. http://jsaldanha.education/_media/

Theo, Sani. (2021, January 8). AI In Aviation: Are You Ready To Fly Without A Human Pilot? | Must Read. Electronics for You. https://www.electronicsforu.com/technology-trends/tech-focus/ai-aviation-fly-without-human-pilot

This Year, Autonomous Trucks Will Take to the Road With No One on Board. (2021). IEEE Spectrum: Technology, Engineering, and Science News. https://spectrum.ieee.org/transportation/self-driving/this-year-autonomous-trucks-will-take-to-the-road-with-no-one-on-board

Using Artificial Intelligence in Cybersecurity | Balbix. (2019, November 27). Balbix. https://www.balbix.com/insights/artificial-intelligence-in-cybersecurity/

Wagner, R. A. (2020, September 11). Informed Consent Form and Important. EMedicineHealth; eMedicineHealth. https://www.emedicinehealth.com/informed_consent/article_em.htm

What is Epidemiology? | Teacher Roadmap. (2021). Centers for Disease Control and Prevention.

https://www.cdc.gov/careerpaths/k12teacherroadmap/epidemiology.html#:~:text=By%20definition%2C%20epidemiology%20is%20the,state%2C%20country%2C%20global).

What jobs are being taken over by robots and computers? (2020). Computer Hope. https://www.computerhope.com/issues/ch001799.htm

Willcocks, L. P., Lacity, M., & Craig, A. (2015). The IT function and robotic process automation - LSE Research Online. Lse.ac.uk. https://doi.org/http://eprints.lse.ac.uk/64519/1/OUWRPS_15_05_published.pdf

Chapter 4 - Brain Computer Interfaces

Ajrawi, S., Rao, R., & Sarkar, M. (2021). Cybersecurity in Brain-Computer Interfaces: RFID-based design-theoretical framework. Informatics in Medicine Unlocked, 22, 100489. https://doi.org/10.1016/j.imu.2020.100489

Aldhaheri, T. A., Kulkarni, S. B., & Bhise, P. R. (2021). Brain-Computer Interfaces and Neurolinguistics: A Short Review. Sustainable Communication Networks and Application, 655–670. https://doi.org/10.1007/978-981-15-8677-4_54

Belkacem, A. N., Jamil, N., Palmer, J. A., Ouhbi, S., & Chen, C. (2020). Brain-Computer Interfaces for Improving the Quality of Life of Older Adults and Elderly Patients. Frontiers in Neuroscience, 14. https://doi.org/10.3389/fnins.2020.00692

Czech, A. (2021). Brain-Computer Interface Use to Control Military Weapons and Tools. Control, Computer Engineering, and Neuroscience, 196–204. https://doi.org/10.1007/978-3-030-72254-8_20

Derksen, M. A. (2021, April). Brain-computer interfaces for people with ataxia: interest, needs and risk acceptance of an overlooked potential user group. https://pure.tue.nl/ws/portalfiles/portal/172827198/Master_Thesis_report_Maxine_Derksen_HTI.pdf

Drew, L. (2019). The ethics of brain-computer interfaces. Nature, 571(7766), S19–S21. https://doi.org/10.1038/d41586-019-02214-2

Gu, X., Cao, Z., Jolfaei, A., Xu, P., Jung, T.-P., & Lin, C.-T. (2015). EEG-based Brain-Computer Interfaces (BCIs): A Survey of Recent Studies on Signal Sensing Technologies and Computational Intelligence Approaches and Their Applications. https://arxiv.org/pdf/2001.11337.pdf

He, B., Yuan, H., Meng, J., & Gao, S. (2020). Brain-Computer Interfaces. Neural Engineering, 131–183. https://doi.org/10.1007/978-3-030-43395-6_4

http://www.brainvision.co.uk/blog/author/admin. (2014, April 30). The Brief History of Brain-Computer Interfaces. Brain Vision UK.

The Brief History of Brain Computer Interfaces - Brain Vision. http://brainvision.co.uk/news-2/the-brief-history-of-brain-computer-interfaces-2.

https://www.facebook.com/NIHAging. (2020). What Are Clinical Trials and Studies? National Institute on Aging. https://www.nia.nih.gov/health/what-are-clinical-trials-and-studies

Kapgate, D. (2020). Future of EEG Based Hybrid Visual Brain-Computer Interface Systems in Rehabilitation of People with Neurological Disorders. International Research Journal on Advanced Science Hub, 2(6), 15–20. https://doi.org/10.47392/irjash.2020.31

Major, A., Wynans, R., Thomas, M., Kiesling, E., Air, M., & Base, F. (2015). MASTER OF OPERATIONAL ARTS AND SCIENCES. https://apps.dtic.mil/sti/pdfs/AD1012768.pdf

Maksimenko, V., Kelderhuis, J., Makarov, V., Innopolis, & Hramov, A. (2020). Brain-computer interface for the epileptic seizures prediction and prevention 1. http://nctech-lab.ru/Content/ArticleImages/50e4bbfe-f8c1-43e2-b26c-671a1273d18d.pdf

Mercado, J., Escobedo, L., & Tentori, M. (2020). A BCI video game using neurofeedback improves the attention of children with autism. Journal on Multimodal User Interfaces, 15(3), 273–281. https://doi.org/10.1007/s12193-020-00339-7

Neural Engineering. (2011). Google Books. https://books.google.ca/books?hl=en&lr=&id=SVZDAAAAQBAJ&oi=fnd&pg=PA87&ots=k1UtoRZGYo&sig=XsL8npUtz_0Tb1jrLV7HhijRZx0#v=onepage&q&f=false

NHS Choices. (2021). Paralysis. https://www.nhs.uk/conditions/paralysis/#:~:text=Paralysis%20is%20the%20loss%20of,may%20be%20temporary%20or%20permanent.

Perry, T. S. (2020, February 25). Here's How Facebook's Brain-Computer Interface Development is Progressing. IEEE Spectrum; IEEE Spectrum. https://spectrum.ieee.org/heres-how-facebooks-braincomputer-interface-development-is-progressing

Ram Sagar. (2021, July 23). Facebook Pulls Plug On Invasive Brain-Machine Interface Research. Analytics India Magazine. https://analyticsindiamag.com/facebook-brain-machine-interface-research-project-steno/#:~:text=Facebook%20Reality%20Labs%20(FRL)%20in,term%20goal%3A%20to%20develop%20a

Roc, A., Pillette, L., Mladenovic, J., Benaroch, C., N'Kaoua, B., Jeunet, C., & Lotte, F. (2021). A review of user training methods in brain-computer interfaces based on mental tasks. Journal of Neural Engineering, 18(1), 011002. https://doi.org/10.1088/1741-2552/abca17

Rouanne, V., Śliwowski, M., Costecalde, T., Benabid, A., & Aksenova, T. (2021). Detection of Error Correlates in the Motor Cortex in a Long Term Clinical Trial of ECoG based Brain-Computer Interface. Proceedings of the 14th International Joint Conference on Biomedical Engineering Systems and Technologies. https://doi.org/10.5220/0010227800260034

Shih, J. J., Krusienski, D. J., & Wolpaw, J. R. (2012). Brain-Computer Interfaces in Medicine. Mayo Clinic Proceedings, 87(3), 268–279. https://doi.org/10.1016/j.mayocp.2011.12.008

World Health Organization: WHO. (2019, June 20). Epilepsy. Who.int; World Health Organization: WHO. https://www.who.int/news-room/fact-sheets/detail/epilepsy#:~:text=Around%2050%20million%20people%20worldwide%20have%20epilepsy%2C%20making%20it%20one,if%20properly%20diagnosed%20and%20treated.

Yu, C.-S., Lin, Y.-J., Lin, C.-H., Lin, S.-Y., Wu, J. L., & Chang, S.-S. (2020). Development of an Online Health Care Assessment for Preventive Medicine: A Machine Learning Approach. Journal of Medical Internet Research, 22(6), e18585. https://doi.org/10.2196/18585

Zeng, Y., Sun, K., & Lu, E. (2021). Declaration on the ethics of brain-computer interfaces and augment intelligence. AI and Ethics, 1(3), 209–211. https://doi.org/10.1007/s43681-020-00036-x

Chapter 5 – Nanomedicine

Astruc D. (2015). Introduction to Nanomedicine. Molecules (Basel, Switzerland), 21(1), E4.

April Cashin-Garbutt, MA (Editor). (2019, January 22). Nanomedicine – Past, Present and Future. Medical News.

Center for Nanomedicine Hopkins. What is Nanomedicine? (2021). The Center for Nanomedicine at Wilmer Eye Institute. Hopkins.

Chaturvedi, V. K., Singh, A., Singh, V. K., & Singh, M. P. (2019). Cancer Nanotechnology: A New Revolution for Cancer Diagnosis and Therapy. Current drug metabolism, 20(6), 416–429. Doi.org.

Cuffari, B. (2018, September 17). Nanotechnology in the USA: Market report. AZoNano.

Dutta, S. S., PhD. (2022, January 18). Nanomedicine and COVID-19. News-Medical.Net. Medical News.

Emergen Research, (2021). Nanotechnology market, by type (nanosensors, Nanodevice, nanomaterials, others), by application (information technology (IT), Homeland Security, medicine, transportation, Food Safety, others), by end-use, and by region forecast to 2030.

Nanotechnology Industry Overview | Nanotechnology Market Forecast by 2030. Emergenresearch.

Engineering and Physical Sciences Research Council (EPSRC). UKRI. (2016). U.K Research and Innovation.

Frequently asked questions. National Nanotechnology Initiative. (2021). Nano.gov.

Future of nanomedicines. ECHA. (2019). Euon.

Gold, Silver, Iron Oxide, Alumina, & amp; Segment Forecasts, 2018 - 2025. Nanomedicine Market Size, Growth | Global Industry Report, 2018-2025. Grandview Research.

MG, K., V, K., & F, H. (2015). History and Possible Uses of Nanomedicine Based on Nanoparticles and Nanotechnological Progress. Journal of Nanomedicine & Nanotechnology, 06(06).

Muthu, M. S., Leong, D. T., Mei, L., & Feng, S. S. (2014). Nanotheranostics - application and further development of nanomedicine strategies for advanced theranostics. Theranostics, 4(6), 660–677.

Nanomedicine Market Analysis By Products (Therapeutics, Regenerative Medicine, Diagnostics), By Application (Clinical Oncology, Infectious diseases), By Nanomolecule.

Nanotechnology in USA | Statnano. (2022.). Drug Products, Including Biological Products, that Contain Nanomaterials; Guidance for Industry 2022. Statnano.

National Nanotechnology Coordination Office (2019). Benefits and Applications. National Nanotechnology Initiative. Nano.gov.

Riehemann, K., Schneider, S., Luger, T., Godin, B., Ferrari, M. and Fuchs, H. (2009), Nanomedicine—Challenge and Perspectives. Angewandte Chemie International Edition, 48: 872-897.

ReportLinker. (2021, January 20). Healthcare nanotechnology (nanomedicine) market - growth, trends, and forecast (2021 - 2026). GlobeNewswire News Room. Globenewswire.

Routley, N. (2019, October 15). The future of nanotechnology in medicine. Visual Capitalist.

Ventola C. L., (2012). The nanomedicine revolution: part 2: current and future clinical applications. P&T: a peer-reviewed journal for formulary management, 37(10), 582–591.

What is Nanomedicine? ETPN. (2021). Nanomedicine.eu.

What is Nanomedicine? Center for Nanomedicine. (2020.). John's Hopkins Medicine.

Chapter 6 - Virtual and Augmented Reality

5 Ways Medical Virtual Reality Is Changing Healthcare. The Medical Futurist. (2020, April 3). https://medicalfuturist.com/5-ways-medical-vr-is-changing-healthcare/.

Anthes, C., Garcia-Hernandez, R. J., Wiedemann, M., & Kranzlmuller, D. (2016). State of the art of virtual reality technology. 2016 IEEE Aerospace Conference. https://doi.org/10.1109/aero.2016.7500674

Arth, C., Graber, L., Grasset, R., Mulloni, A., Schmalstieg, D., & Wagner, D. (2015). The History of Mobile Augmented Reality. Inst. for Computer Graphics and Vision Graz University of Technology, Austria.

Ayoub, A., & Pulijala, Y. (2019). The application of virtual reality and augmented reality in Oral & Maxillofacial Surgery. BMC Oral Health, 19(1). https://doi.org/10.1186/s12903-019-0937-8

Aziz, H. A. (2018). Virtual Reality Programs Applications in Healthcare. Journal of Health & Medical Informatics, 09(01). https://doi.org/10.4172/2157-7420.1000305

Bestsennyy, O., Gilbert, G., Harris, A., & Rost, J. (2021, July 14). Telehealth: A quarter-trillion-dollar post-COVID-19 reality? McKinsey & Company. https://www.mckinsey.com/industries/healthcare-systems-and-services/our-insights/telehealth-a-quarter-trillion-dollar-post-covid-19-reality.

Breining, G. (2018, August 28). Future or fad? Virtual reality in medical education. AAMC. https://www.aamc.org/news-insights/future-or-fad-virtual-reality-medical-education.

CHARIOT Program. Stanford Children's Health. (2018). https://www.stanfordchildrens.org/en/innovation/chariot.

Chen, Y., Wang, Q., Chen, H., Song, X., Tang, H., & Tian, M. (2019). An overview of augmented reality technology. Journal of Physics: Conference Series, 1237, 022082. https://doi.org/10.1088/1742-6596/1237/2/022082

Feng, H., Li, C., Liu, J., Wang, L., Ma, J., Li, G., Gan, L., Shang, X., & Wu, Z. (2019). Virtual Reality Rehabilitation Versus Conventional Physical Therapy for Improving Balance and Gait in Parkinson's Disease Patients: A Randomized Controlled Trial. Medical Science Monitor, 25, 4186–4192. https://doi.org/10.12659/msm.916455

García-Betances, R. I., Jiménez-Mixco, V., Arredondo, M. T., & Cabrera-Umpiérrez, M. F. (2014). Using Virtual Reality for Cognitive Training of the Elderly. American Journal of Alzheimer's Disease & Other Dementiasr, 30(1), 49–54. https://doi.org/10.1177/1533317514545866

Haptic – Adding a New Dimension to Virtual Reality. FutureBridge. (2020, May 20). https://www.futurebridge.com/industry/perspectives-mobility/haptic-adding-a-new-dimension-to-virtual-reality/.

Huang, T.-K., Yang, C.-H., Hsieh, Y.-H., Wang, J.-C., & Hung, C.-C. (2018). Augmented reality (AR) and virtual reality (VR) applied in dentistry. The Kaohsiung Journal of Medical Sciences, 34(4), 243–248. https://doi.org/10.1016/j.kjms.2018.01.009

Matthews, K. (2021, June 10). 18 Healthcare Augmented Reality and Virtual Reality Companies to Watch. Healthcare IT News. https://hitconsultant.net/2020/06/29/augmented-reality-and-virtual-reality-companies-to-watch/#.YPXikmhKhPa.

Mazuryk , T., & Gervautz, M. (1999). Tomasz Mazuryk and Michael Gervautz. Institute of Computer Graphics Vienna University of Technology, Austria.

Muinga, N., & Paton, C. (2019). Virtual Reality for Medical and Nursing Training in Low- and Middle-Income Countries. Pathways for Prosperity Commission Background Paper Series, 25.

Rizzo, A. 'S., & Shilling, R. (2017). Clinical Virtual Reality tools to advance the prevention, assessment, and treatment of PTSD. European Journal of Psychotraumatology, 8(sup5), 1414560. https://doi.org/10.1080/20008198.2017.1414560

Rizzo, A., Schultheis, M., & Rothbaum, B. (2003). ETHICAL ISSUES FOR THE USE OF VIRTUAL REALITY IN THE PSYCHOLOGICAL SCIENCES. Swets & Zeitlinger Publishers.

Sik-Lanyi, C. (2017). Virtual reality healthcare system could be a potential future of health consultations. 2017 IEEE 30th Neumann Colloquium (NC). https://doi.org/10.1109/nc.2017.8263275

Sutherland, J., Belec, J., Sheikh, A., Chepelev, L., Althobaity, W., Chow, B. J., Mitsouras, D., Christensen, A., Rybicki, F. J., & La Russa, D. J. (2018). Applying Modern Virtual and Augmented Reality Technologies to Medical Images and Models. Journal of Digital Imaging, 32(1), 38–53. https://doi.org/10.1007/s10278-018-0122-7

United Nations. (2020). Ageing and disability Enable. United Nations. https://www.un.org/development/desa/disabilities/disability-and-ageing.html.

Verhey, J. T., Haglin, J. M., Verhey, E. M., & Hartigan, D. E. (2020). Virtual, augmented, and mixed reality applications in orthopedic surgery. The International Journal of Medical Robotics and Computer Assisted Surgery, 16(2). https://doi.org/10.1002/rcs.2067

Wang, Y.-J., Chen, P.-J., Liang, X., & Lin, Y.-H. (2017). Augmented reality with image registration, vision correction and sunlight readability via liquid crystal devices. Scientific Reports, 7(1). https://doi.org/10.1038/s41598-017-00492-2

Wiederhold, B. K., & Riva, G. (2019). Virtual Reality Therapy: Emerging Topics and Future Challenges. Cyberpsychology, Behavior, and Social Networking, 22(1), 3–6. https://doi.org/10.1089/cyber.2018.29136.bkw

Chapter 7 - Robotics and Robot-Assisted Surgery

5 medical robots making a difference in healthcare at CWRU. at CWRU. (2020). https://online-engineering.case.edu/blog/medical-robots-making-a-difference.

Alaiad, A., & Zhou, L. (2014). The determinants of home healthcare robots adoption: An empirical investigation. International Journal of Medical Informatics, 83(11), 825–840. https://doi.org/10.1016/j.ijmedinf.2014.07.003

Alonzo, I. (2020, August 27). Breakthrough! these tiny robots can enter your bloodstream and perform microsurgery! Tech Times. https://www.techtimes.com/articles/252069/20200826/scientists-invent-micro-robots-surgery-medical-field-breakthrough-enter-through.htm.

Archibald, M. M., & Barnard, A. (2017). Futurism in nursing: Technology, robotics and the fundamentals of care. Journal of Clinical Nursing, 27(11-12), 2473–2480. https://doi.org/10.1111/jocn.14081

Ashley, S. (2017, May 30). Robotic exoskeletons are changing lives in surprising ways. NBCNews.com. https://www.nbcnews.com/mach/innovation/robotic-exoskeletons-are-changing-lives-surprising-ways-n722676.

BBC. (2020). What the world can learn from Japan's robots. BBC Worklife. https://www.bbc.com/worklife/article/20200205-what-the-world-can-learn-from-japans-robots.

Begić, A. (2018). Application of service robots FOR disinfection in medical institutions. Lecture Notes in Networks and Systems, 1056–1065. https://doi.org/10.1007/978-3-319-71321-2_89

Blake, E. A., Sheeder, J., Behbakht, K., Guntupalli, S. R., & Guy, M. S. (2016). Factors impacting use of robotic surgery for treatment of endometrial cancer in the United States. Annals of Surgical Oncology, 23(11), 3744–3748. https://doi.org/10.1245/s10434-016-5252-x

Brodie, A., & Vasdev, N. (2018). The future of robotic surgery. The Annals of The Royal College of Surgeons of England, 100(Supplement 7), 4–13. https://doi.org/10.1308/rcsann.supp2.4

Bulboacă, A. E., Bolboacă, S. D., & Bulboacă, A. C. (2017). Ethical considerations in providing an upper limb exoskeleton device for stroke patients. Medical Hypotheses, 101, 61–64. https://doi.org/10.1016/j.mehy.2017.02.016

Chen, K., Lou, V. W.-qun, Tan, K. C.-kian, Wai, M.-yi, & Chan, L.-lok. (2020). Effects of a humanoid companion robot on dementia symptoms and caregiver distress for residents in long-term care. Journal of the American Medical Directors Association, 21(11). https://doi.org/10.1016/j.jamda.2020.05.036

Denning, N.-L., Kallis, M. P., & Prince, J. M. (2020). Pediatric robotic surgery. Surgical Clinics of North America, 100(2), 431–443. https://doi.org/10.1016/j.suc.2019.12.004

Geiger, J. D., & Hirschl, R. B. (2015). Innovation in surgical technology and techniques: Challenges and ethical issues. Seminars in Pediatric Surgery, 24(3), 115–121. https://doi.org/10.1053/j.sempedsurg.2015.02.008

George, E. I., Brand, T. C., LaPorta, A., Marescaux, J., & Satava, R. M. (2018). Origins of robotic surgery: From skepticism to standard of care. JSLS : Journal of the Society of Laparoendoscopic Surgeons, 22(4). https://doi.org/10.4293/jsls.2018.00039

Gyles, C. (2019). Robots in medicine. The Canadian Veterinary Journal. https://www.ncbi.nlm.nih.gov/pmc/articles/PMC6625162/.

Hockstein, N. G., Gourin, C. G., Faust, R. A., & Terris, D. J. (2007). A history of robots: From science fiction to surgical robotics. Journal of Robotic Surgery, 1(2), 113–118. https://doi.org/10.1007/s11701-007-0021-2

Ishikawa, N., & Watanabe, G. (2015). Robot-Assisted cardiac surgery. Annals of Thoracic and Cardiovascular Surgery, 21(4), 322–328. https://doi.org/10.5761/atcs.ra.15-00145

Jara, R. D., Guerrón, A. D., & Portenier, D. (2020). Complications of robotic surgery. Surgical Clinics of North America, 100(2), 461–468. https://doi.org/10.1016/j.suc.2019.12.008

Jimmy Rose. (2015, June 2). This autonomous medical robot can assist nurses. ExtremeTech. https://www.extremetech.com/extreme/207130-terapio-autonomous-medical-robot-can-assist-nurses.

Jin, L. X., Ibrahim, A. M., Newman, N. A., Makarov, D. V., Pronovost, P. J., & Makary, M. A. (2011). Robotic surgery claims on United States hospital websites. Journal for Healthcare Quality, 33(6), 48–52. https://doi.org/10.1111/j.1945-1474.2011.00148.x

Jin, L. X., Ibrahim, A. M., Newman, N. A., Makarov, D. V., Pronovost, P. J., & Makary, M. A. (2011). Robotic surgery claims on United States hospital websites. Journal for Healthcare Quality, 33(6), 48–52. https://doi.org/10.1111/j.1945-1474.2011.00148.x

Kalan, S., Chauhan, S., Coelho, R. F., Orvieto, M. A., Camacho, I. R., Palmer, K. J., & Patel, V. R. (2010). History of robotic surgery. Journal of Robotic Surgery, 4(3), 141–147. https://doi.org/10.1007/s11701-010-0202-2

Kaushik, D., High, R., Clark, C. J., & LaGrange, C. A. (2010). Malfunction of the da Vinci robotic system During Robot-assisted LAPAROSCOPIC prostatectomy: An international survey. Journal of Endourology, 24(4), 571–575. https://doi.org/10.1089/end.2009.0489

Louie, D. R., & Eng, J. J. (2016). Powered robotic exoskeletons in post-stroke rehabilitation of gait: A scoping review. Journal of NeuroEngineering and Rehabilitation, 13(1). https://doi.org/10.1186/s12984-016-0162-5

Louie, D. R., & Eng, J. J. (2016). Powered robotic exoskeletons in post-stroke rehabilitation of gait: A scoping review. Journal of NeuroEngineering and Rehabilitation, 13(1). https://doi.org/10.1186/s12984-016-0162-5

Matthews, K. (2019, December 5). The growing emergence of robots in HEALTHCARE: Key opportunities & benefits. The Growing Emergence of Robots in Healthcare: Opportunities & Benefits. https://hitconsultant.net/2019/12/05/the-growing-emergence-of-robots-in-healthcare-key-opportunities-benefits/#.YQLkiWhKhPY.

Mayo Foundation for Medical Education and Research. (2021, March 26). Robotic surgery. Mayo Clinic. https://www.mayoclinic.org/tests-procedures/robotic-surgery/about/pac-20394974#:~:text=Robotic%20surgery%20is%20usually%20associated,certain%20traditional%20open%20surgical%20procedures.

McDonnell, J. M., Ahern, D. P., Ó Doinn, T., Gibbons, D., Rodrigues, K. N., Birch, N., & Butler, J. S. (2020). Surgeon proficiency in robot-assisted spine surgery. The Bone & Joint Journal, 102-B(5), 568–572. https://doi.org/10.1302/0301-620x.102b5.bjj-2019-1392.r2

Murphy, D., Challacombe, B., Khan, M. S., & Dasgupta, P. (2006). Robotic technology in urology. Postgraduate Medical Journal, 82(973), 743–747. https://doi.org/10.1136/pgmj.2006.048140

Rakhymbayeva, N., Amirova, A., & Sandygulova, A. (2021). A long-term engagement with a social robot for autism therapy. Frontiers in Robotics and AI, 8. https://doi.org/10.3389/frobt.2021.669972

Ruhle, B. C., Ferguson Bryan, A., & Grogan, R. H. (2019). Robot-Assisted endocrine SURGERY: Indications and drawbacks. Journal of Laparoendoscopic & Advanced Surgical Techniques, 29(2), 129–135. https://doi.org/10.1089/lap.2018.0308

Schmidt, C. K., Medina-Sánchez, M., Edmondson, R. J., & Schmidt, O. G. (2020). Engineering microrobots for targeted cancer therapies from a medical perspective. Nature Communications, 11(1). https://doi.org/10.1038/s41467-020-19322-7

Shen, T., Afsar, M. R., Zhang, H., Ye, C., & Shen, X. (2020). A 3D Computer Vision-Guided Robotic companion FOR Non-Contact human assistance and rehabilitation. Journal of Intelligent & Robotic Systems, 100(3-4), 911–923. https://doi.org/10.1007/s10846-020-01258-1

Small wonders: Microbots in medicine and engineering. Orange Business Services. (2018, October 8). https://www.orange-business.com/en/blogs/small-wonders-microbots-medicine-and-engineering.

The top 12 social companion robots. The Medical Futurist. (2020, March 16). https://medicalfuturist.com/the-top-12-social-companion-robots/.

Yang, G.-Z., J. Nelson, B., Murphy, R. R., Choset, H., Christensen, H., H. Collins, S., Dario, P., Goldberg, K., Ikuta, K., Jacobstein, N., Kragic, D., Taylor, R. H., & McNutt, M. (2020). Combating covid-19—the role of robotics in managing public health and infectious diseases. Science Robotics, 5(40). https://doi.org/10.1126/scirobotics.abb5589

Chapter 8 - 3D Printing

3D printing in healthcare - the future of healthcare is here. Tractus3D. (2022). https://tractus3d.com/used-by/branches/healthcare/.

3D Printing in Healthcare: Healthcare Trends. Pharmaceutical Technology. (2022). https://www.pharmaceutical-technology.com/comment/3d-printing-healthcare/.

3D Printing Medical Devices Market Size, Industry, Analysis & Forecast. Verified Market Research. (2022). https://www.verifiedmarketresearch.com/product/3d-printing-medical-devices-market/.

Arun H. Healthcare 3D Printing Market 2018 Prominent Players-Aprecia Pharmaceuticals.

ASTM. Standard Technology for Additive Manufacturing-General Principles/Terminology. West Conshohocken, PA, USA: ASTM ISO/ASTM 52900:2015 (E); 2015.

Aspect Biosystems, Bio 3D Technologies, Biobots, Cyfuse Biomedical, Digilab, 3 Dynamics Systems, Envision Tec, Luxexcel, Materialise NV, Nano 3D Biosciences, Oceanz, Organovo Ho. openPR.com

Bastawrous, Wu, L., Strzelecki, B., Levin, D. B., Li, J.-S., Coburn, J., & Ripley, B. (2021). Establishing Quality and Safety in Hospital-based 3D Printing Programs: Patient-first Approach. Radiographics, 41(4), 1208–1229. https://doi.org/10.1148/rg.2021200175.

Chaudhuri, Naseraldin, H., Søberg, P. V., Kroll, E., & Librus, M. (2020). Should hospitals invest in customized on-demand 3D printing for surgeries? International Journal of Operations & Production Management, 41(1), 55–62. https://doi.org/10.1108/IJOPM-05-2020-0277.

Cohen A., Laviv A., Berman P., Nashef R., Abu-Tair J. Mandibular reconstruction using stereolithographic 3-dimensional printing modeling technology. Oral Surgery, Oral Medicine,

Oral Pathology, Oral Radiology, and Endodontology. 2009;108(5):661–666. doi: 10.1016/j.tripleo.2009.05.023.

Diment L. E., Thompson M. S., Bergmann J. H. M. Clinical efficacy and effectiveness of 3D printing: a systematic review. BMJ Open. 2017;7(12) doi: 10.1136/bmjopen-2017-016891.e016891

Grand View Research. (2022). Healthcare 3D Printing Market Analysis By Application (Surgical Guides, Implants, Surgical Instruments, Bioengineering), By Technology (Electron Beam Melting, Stereolithography, Droplet Deposition Manufacturing), By Raw Material (Metals, Biological Cells, Polymers, Ceramics) And Segment Forecast to 2020. San Francisco: Grand View Research.

Jovic, T., Combellack, E., Jessop, Z., & Whitaker, I. (2020). 3D Bioprinting and the Future of Surgery. Frontiers In Surgery, 7. https://doi.org/10.3389/fsurg.2020.609836

Mazher I. M., Angus P. F., Santosh K. M., Gibson I. Customised design and development of patient-specific 3D printed whole mandible implant. Proceedings of the 27th Annual International Solid Freeform Fabrication Symposium; August 2016; Austin, TX, USA.

Mondschein R. J., Kanitkar A., Williams C. B., Verbridge S. S., Long T. E. Polymer structure-property requirements for stereolithographic 3D printing of soft tissue engineering scaffolds. Biomaterials. 2017;140:170–188. doi: 10.1016/j.biomaterials.2017.06.005.

Pillai, Upadhyay, A., Khayambashi, P., Farooq, I., Sabri, H., Tarar, M., Lee, K. T., Harb, I., Zhou, S., Wang, Y., & Tran, S. D. (2021). Dental 3D-Printing: Transferring Art from the Laboratories to the Clinics. Polymers, 13(1), 157. https://doi.org/10.3390/polym13010157.

Phan K., Sgro A., Maharaj M. M., D'Urso P., Mobbs R. J. Application of a 3D custom printed patient-specific spinal implant for C1/2 arthrodesis. Journal of Spine Surgery. 2016;2(4):314–318. doi: 10.21037/jss.2016.12.06.

Shafiee, & Atala, A. (2016). Printing Technologies for Medical Applications. Trends in Molecular Medicine, 22(3), 254–265. https://doi.org/10.1016/j.molmed.2016.01.003.

Ventola C. L. Medical applications for 3D printing: current and projected uses. Pharmacy and Therapeutics. 2014;39(10):704–711.

Whitley D., Eidson R. S., Rudek I., Bencharit S. In-office fabrication of dental implant surgical guides using desktop stereolithographic printing and implant treatment planning software: a clinical report. Journal of Prosthetic Dentistry. 2017;118(3):256–263.

Zhu W., Ma X., Gou M., Mei D., Zhang K., Chen S. 3D printing of functional biomaterials for tissue engineering. Current opinion in biotechnology. 2016;40:103–112. doi: 10.1016/j.copbio.2016.03.014.

Chapter 9 - Healthcare Trackers, Wearables, and Sensors

A Study of Fitness Trackers and Wearables. (January 2021). https://www.hfe.co.uk/blog/a-study-of-fitness-trackers-and-wearables/

Are Currently Available Wearable Devices for Activity Tracking and Heart Rate Monitoring Accurate, Precise, and Medically Beneficial?. (2021). https://synapse.koreamed.org/articles/1075768

Breast Cancer Survivors' Experiences With an Activity Tracker Integrated Into a Supervised Exercise Program: Qualitative Study. (2019). https://pubmed.ncbi.nlm.nih.gov/30789349/

Can a Free Wearable Activity Tracker Change Behavior? (2022). https://www.researchprotocols.org/2016/4/e237/

Diabetes Educators' Insights Regarding Connecting Mobile Phone– and Wearable Tracker–Collected Self-Monitoring Information to a Nationally-Used Electronic Health Record System for Diabetes Education: Descriptive Qualitative Study. (2019). https://mhealth.jmir.org/2018/7/e10206/

Doctors monitor patients remotely via smartphones and fitness trackers. (April 2021.). https://www.pbs.org/newshour/health/doctors-monitor-patients-vitals-via-smartphones-fitness-trackers

Evolution of Wearable Devices with Real-Time Disease Monitoring. (July 2021). https://www.ncbi.nlm.nih.gov/pmc/articles/PMC6631918/

Impact of remote patient monitoring on clinical outcomes: An updated meta-analysis of randomized controlled trials. (2020). https://www.nature.com/articles/s41746-017-0002-4

Increasing Patient Engagement Through the Use of Wearable Technology. (2020). https://www.npjournal.org/article/S1555-4155(18)31275-3/pdf

Medical Education - The Medical Futurist. (2020). https://medicalfuturist.com/category/medical-education/

Patients' experiences with commercially available activity trackers embedded in physiotherapy treatment: A qualitative study. (2021). https://www.tandfonline.com/doi/full/10.1080/09638288.2019.1590470

Sensors in medicine. (2022). https://www.ncbi.nlm.nih.gov/pmc/articles/PMC1129066/

Smart Sensors for Healthcare and Medical Applications. (2020). https://www.ncbi.nlm.nih.gov/pmc/articles/PMC7828709/

The dark side of wearables: How they're secretly jeopardizing your security and privacy. (March 2021). https://www.techrepublic.com/index.php/article/the-dark-side-of-wearables-how-theyre-secretly-jeopardizing-your-security-and-privacy/

The Future of Wearable Technologies and Remote Monitoring in Health Care. (2021). https://ascopubs.org/doi/full/10.1200/EDBK_238919

Use and Adoption Challenges of Wearable Activity Trackers. (2021). https://www.ideals.illinois.edu/bitstream/handle/2142/73649/164_ready.pdf

Use of menstruation and fertility app trackers: a scoping review of the evidence (2019). https://srh.bmj.com/content/47/2/90

Using an Activity Tracker in Healthcare: Experiences of Healthcare Professionals and Patients. (2018). https://www.mdpi.com/1660-4601/18/10/5147/htm

Wearable sensors can tell when you are getting sick | Stanford Medicine News Center. (2019). https://med.stanford.edu/news/all-news/2017/01/wearable-sensors-can-tell-when-you-are-getting-sick.html

Wearable Tech in Healthcare: Possibilities and Pitfalls | HealthTech .. (2020). https://healthtechmagazine.net/article/2021/04/wearable-tech-healthcare-possibilities-and-pitfalls-perfcon

Wearable Technology Applications in Healthcare: A Literature Review. (2018). https://www.himss.org/resources/wearable-technology-applications-healthcare-literature-review

Wearable Technology for Cardiology: An Update and Framework for the Future. (2018). https://www.ncbi.nlm.nih.gov/pmc/articles/PMC5762264/

Wearables and the medical revolution | Personalized Medicine. (2021). https://www.futuremedicine.com/doi/10.2217/pme-2018-0044

What You Need to Know About Health Tracking | UIC Online Health .. (February 2021). https://healthinformatics.uic.edu/blog/what-you-need-to-know-about-health-tracking/

Chapter 10 Medical Tricorder

Amisha, Malik, P., Pathania, M., & Rathaur, V. K. (2019). Overview of artificial intelligence in medicine. Journal of Family Medicine and Primary Care, 8(7), 2328. https://doi.org/10.4103/jfmpc.jfmpc_440_19

Basu, S., Phillips, R. S., Berkowitz, S. A., Landon, B. E., Bitton, A., & Phillips, R. L. (2021). Estimated Effect on Life Expectancy of Alleviating Primary Care Shortages in the United States. Annals of Internal Medicine, 174(7), 920–926. https://doi.org/10.7326/m20-7381

Bennock, S. (2017, March 3). Resilience in Positive Psychology: Bouncing Back & Staying Strong. https://positivepsychology.com/resilience-in-positive-psychology/

Could DX. (2021). Vitaliti. clouddx.com. https://www.clouddx.com/#/vitaliti.

DxtER™. Basil Leaf Technologies. (2020). http://www.basilleaftech.com/dxter.

Dynamical Biomarkers Group: Qualcomm Tricorder XPRIZE. Dynamical Biomarkers Group | Qualcomm Tricorder XPRIZE. (2021).

Empowering personal healthcare. XPRIZE. (2020). https://www.xprize.org/prizes/tricorder.

MEDICAL TRICORDERS ARE REAL. SERIOUSLY. XPRIZE. (2017). https://www.xprize.org/articles/medical-tricorders-are-real-seriously.

DxtER™. Basil Leaf Technologies. (2021). http://www.basilleaftech.com/dxter.

Could DX. (2021). Vitaliti. clouddx.com. https://www.clouddx.com/#/vitaliti.

Family-led team takes top prize in qualcomm tricorder xprize. XPRIZE. (2019). https://www.xprize.org/prizes/tricorder/articles/family-led-team-takes-top-prize-in-qualcomm-tricor.

ForeSee Medical, Inc. (2018). Medical Algorithms For Treatment & Diagnostic Testing. ForeSee Medical. https://www.foreseemed.com/medical-algorithms#:~:text=There%20are%20many%20algorithms%20in,reduce%20the%20possibility%20of%20errors.

Ledford, H. (2019, October 24). Millions of black people affected by racial bias in health-care algorithms. Nature News. https://www.nature.com/articles/d41586-019-03228-6.

Netflix, Inc. (2020). The Social Dilemma. https://www.netflix.com/title/81254224.

Mann, D. M., Chen, J., Chunara, R., Testa, P. A., & Nov, O. (2020). COVID-19 transforms health care through telemedicine: Evidence from the field. Journal of the American Medical Informatics Association, 27(7), 1132–1135. https://doi.org/10.1093/jamia/ocaa072

MedWand Solutions, Inc. (2017). Technology. MedWand. https://medwand.com/technology.html.

MEDICAL TRICORDERS ARE REAL. SERIOUSLY. XPRIZE.. https://www.xprize.org/articles/medical-tricorders-are-real-seriously.

Miner, H. (1956). Body Ritual among the Nacirema. AnthroSource. https://anthrosource.onlinelibrary.wiley.com/action/showCitFormats?doi=10.1525%2Faa.1956.58.3.02a00080.

Pahar, M., Klopper, M., Warren, R., & Niesler, T. (2021). COVID-19 cough classification using machine learning and global smartphone recordings. Computers in biology and medicine, 135, 104572. Advance online publication. https://doi.org/10.1016/j.compbiomed.2021.104572

Rasmus, D. (2017, May 30). Star Trek's Tricorder, realized? This device uses AI to diagnose medical conditions. GeekWire. https://www.geekwire.com/2017/star-treks-tricorder-realized-device-uses-ai-diagnose-medical-conditions

Roosevelt Capital Group. (2021, March 31). FILING STATEMENT IN RESPECT OF THE QUALIFYING TRANSACTION OF ROOSEVELT CAPITAL GROUP INC. INVOLVING THE ARRANGEMENT OF CLOUD DX, INC. AND 12632926 CANADA LTD. AND 12686163 CANADA INC. https://sec.report/otc/financial-report/287977

The Economist Newspaper. (2012, December 1). The dream of the medical tricorder. The Economist. https://www.economist.com/technology-quarterly/2012/12/01/the-dream-of-the-medical-tricorder.

Uyeda, J. (2011, August 22). Lasting evolutionary change takes about one million years. Life at OSU. https://today.oregonstate.edu/archives/2011/aug/lasting-evolutionary-change-takes-about-one-million-years.

World Health Organization. (2021). Tuberculosis (TB). World Health Organization. https://www.who.int/news-room/fact-sheets/detail/tuberculosis.

XPrize FAQs. DBIOM. (2021). https://dbiom.org/xprize/faqs#faqnoanchor.

YouTube. (2020). Star Trek, the Qualcomm Tricorder Xprize, and the Future of Medicine (part 1 of 2). YouTube. https://www.youtube.com/watch?v=ssxRivT3c90.

XPrize FAQs. DBIOM. (2020). https://dbiom.org/xprize/faqs#faqnoanchor.

YouTube. (2018). We're Getting Closer to Real-Life Tricorders. YouTube. https://www.youtube.com/watch?v=u28mG226k-A.

Chapter 11 - Genome Sequencing and Editing

Careers in Medical Genetics. (2021). American College of Medical Genetics and Genomics.https://www.acmg.net/ACMG/ACMG/Education/Student/Careers_in_Medical_Genetics.aspx.

Carrier Screening. (2020, December). American College of Obstetricians and Gynecologists. https://www.acog.org/womens-health/faqs/carrier-screening.

DNA Sequencing. (9 November 2021). Testing.com. https://www.testing.com/dna-sequencing/.

DNA Sequencing Fact Sheet. (16 August 2020). National Human Genome Research Institute. https://www.genome.gov/about-genomics/fact-sheets/DNA-Sequencing-Fact-Sheet.

Genetic Engineering. (2021). BBC. https://www.bbc.co.uk/bitesize/guides/zqqs2nb/revision/1.

Genetic Testing. (23 March 2020). Centers for Disease Control and Prevention. https://www.cdc.gov/genomics/gtesting/genetic_testing.htm.

Green, E., Rubin, E., Olson, M. (12 October 2017). The future of DNA sequencing. Macmillan Publishers Limited. https://www.nature.com/articles/550179a.pdf.

Heather, James M., Chain, Benjamin. (10 November 2015). The sequence of sequencers: The history of sequencing DNA. Elsevier.

How Doctors Use Genomics. (2021). Cincinnati Children's. https://www.cincinnatichildrens.org/research/divisions/c/genomics/patients-families/doctors-genomics.

How does DNA Sequencing Work? (2004). Genome News Network. http://www.genomenewsnetwork.org/resources/whats_a_genome/Chp2_2.shtml.

Lung Cancer Genomic Testing. (2021). Memorial Sloan Kettering Cancer Center. https://www.mskcc.org/cancer-care/types/lung/diagnosis/genetic-testing.

Mardis, Elaine R. (5 January 2017). DNA Sequencing Technologies: 2006-2016. Nature Protocols. https://www.nature.com/articles/nprot.2016.182.

Scott, Andrew. (8 March 2018). A CRISPR path to drug discovery. Macmillan Publishers Limited.

https://media.nature.com/original/magazine-assets/d41586-018-02477-1/d41586-018-02477-1.pdf.

Waltz, Emily. (3 May 2021). First genetically-modified mosquitoes released in the United States. Nature. https://www.nature.com/articles/d41586-021-01186-6.

Weil, Alan R. (May 2018). Precision Medicine. People-to-People Health Foundation.

https://www.healthaffairs.org/doi/pdf/10.1377/hlthaff.2018.0520?url_ver=Z39.88-2003&rfr_id=ori%Arid%3Acrossref.org&rfr_dat=cr_pub++0pubmed.

What are genome editing and CRISPR-Cas9? (18 September 2020). Medline Plus. https://medlineplus.gov/genetics/understanding/genomicresearch/genomeediting/.

What is Next Generation DNA Sequencing? (2019) European Molecular Biology Laboratory. https://www.ebi.ac.uk/training/online/courses/functional-genomics-ii-common-technologies-and-daa-analysis-methods/next-generation-sequencing/.

Chapter 12 - New Drug Developments

A historical overview of drug discovery. (2020). https://pubmed.ncbi.nlm.nih.gov/20694682/

Back to the future: Psychedelic drugs in psychiatry - Harvard Health. (2017). https://www.health.harvard.edu/blog/back-to-the-future-psychedelic-drugs-in-psychiatry-202106222508

Drug Development - an overview | ScienceDirect Topics. (2021). https://www.sciencedirect.com/topics/nursing-and-health-professions/drug-development

Drug Development Challenges - NCBI - NIH. (2020). https://www.ncbi.nlm.nih.gov/books/NBK195047/

Future of Pharma & the Pharmaceutical Industry. (2021). https://medicalfuturist.com/category/future-of-pharma/

History of drug discovery and development - UC Davis. (2020). http://scalettar.physics.ucdavis.edu/frs/historyofdrugdiscovery1.pdf

Medicines in Development | PhRMA. (2019). https://www.phrma.org/Science/In-The-Pipeline/Medicines-in-Development

Opportunities and Challenges for Drug Development: Public–Private Partnerships, Adaptive Designs and Big Data. (2020). https://www.frontiersin.org/articles/10.3389/fphar.2016.00461/full

Prescription Medicines | National Institute on Drug Abuse (NIDA). (2020). https://www.drugabuse.gov/drug-topics/prescription-medicines

Pros and Cons of Pharmaceutical Drugs - CUNY Baruch College. (2021). https://blogs.baruch.cuny.edu/herbalandpharmaceuticalmedices/?page_id=16

The drug development process, fda.gov. (2021). https://www.fda.gov/patients/learn-about-drug-and-device-approvals/drug-development-process

The Future of Pharma: The Role Of Biotech Companies. (2019). https://www.forbes.com/sites/forbestechcouncil/2019/05/29/the-future-of-pharma-the-role-of-biotech-companies/

The Importance of Clinical Trials in Drug Development. (2020). https://www.ncbi.nlm.nih.gov/pmc/articles/PMC5124250/

The Importance of Discovering New Drugs. (2018). https://www.azolifesciences.com/article/The-Importance-of-Discovering-New-Drugs.aspx

Therapeutic Drug Use - National Center for Health Statistics. (2021). https://www.cdc.gov/nchs/fastats/drug-use-therapeutic.htm

Think It Through: Managing the Benefits and Risks of Medicines | FDA. (2018). https://www.fda.gov/drugs/information-consumers-and-patients-drugs/think-it-through-managing-benefits-and-risks-medicines

This is how the pharmaceutical industry will look like in 2030. (2017). https://fifarma.org/en/this-is-how-the-pharmaceutical-industry-will-look-like-in-2030/

Understanding Medicines and What They Do - Kids Health. (2019). https://kidshealth.org/en/teens/meds.html

What are the drugs of the future? (2020). https://www.ncbi.nlm.nih.gov/pmc/articles/PMC6072476/

What to expect from the next decade of drug development. (2018). https://www.weforum.org/agenda/2020/02/technology-in-drug-discovery-and-development/

What Will the Pharma World Look Like in 2050? (2017). https://globalforum.diaglobal.org/issue/august-2018/what-will-the-pharma-world-look-like-in-2050/

www.ingramcontent.com/pod-product-compliance
Lightning Source LLC
LaVergne TN
LVHW052302200926
848481LV00002B/439
* 9 7 9 8 2 3 3 7 7 6 5 4 0 *